A RE-APPRAISAL of PATANJALI'S YOGA-SUTRAS

in the light of

THE BUDDHA'S TEACHING

Vipassana Research Institute
Dhamma Giri, Igatpuri 422 403

E17 - A RE-APPRAISAL of PATANJALI'S YOGA-SUTRAS

First Edition : May 1995
Second Edition : 2005
Reprint : 2007, 2011, Dec. 2015

Price: Rs. 96.00

ISBN 81-7414-024-7

Published by:
Vipassana Research Institute
Dhamma Giri, Igatpuri 422 403
Dist. Nashik, Maharashtra, India
Tel: [91] (2553) 244076, 244086, 243712,
243238; Fax: [91] (2553) 244176
Email: vri_admin@dhamma.net.in
info@giri.dhamma.org
Website : www.vridhamma.org

Printed by:
Apollo Printing Press
G-259, SICOF Ltd., 69 MIDC, Satpur
Nashik-422007, Maharashtra

A RE-APPRAISAL OF PATANJALI'S YOGA-SUTRAS

CONTENTS

PREFACE

Patanjali is reputed to be the author of the treatise popularly known as the Yoga-Sutras (Aphorisms on Yoga). An Indian tradition[1] identifies him with the author of the Mahābhāṣya[2]—his namesake—who lived in the 2nd century B.C. as a priest of the ruler Puṣyamitra of the Śuṅga dynasty.

Siddhārtha Gotama the Buddha, who lived in the 6th century B.C., preceded Patanjali by a few centuries. His teaching left a very deep impression on the minds of the suffering humanity with the result that a very large number of people began to follow the path he prescribed. This required observance of certain precepts of morality, practice of concentration of mind and insight-meditation.[3]

Asoka, the great emperor of India whose empire flourished in the 3rd century B.C., himself benefited immensely from the teaching of the Buddha and made it a mission of his life to spread it to the neighbouring countries and abroad. As a result of his efforts, millions of people took to the practice of insight-meditation which enabled them to come out of their suffering and live a life of real peace and harmony.

When Patanjali undertook to compose the Yoga-Sutras there was considerable influence of the Buddha's teaching on the public mind. Obviously he (or, for that matter, anyone else) could not think of going ahead with such a composition without incorporating in it the essentials of the existing practice with which the people had become quite familiar. It is for this reason that the Yoga-Sutras exhibit considerable influence of the Buddha's teaching, although some influence of

---

1. also believed by some western scholars like Lossen and Garbe.
2. the 'Great Gloss' on Pāṇini's Sūtras (a grammatical work of exceptional merit).
3. known as *'sīla'* (सील), *'samādhi'* (समाधि) and *'paññā'* (पञ्ञा).

the Sāṅkhya tenets is also discernible while the innovations made by the author himself are quite obvious.[1]

On all accounts, Patanjali can be said to be a codifier of what was considered by him to be the best in his times in the realm of meditation. About his composition Prof. A.B. Keith,[2] however, remarks: "It is a confused text which is only intelligible by the aid of the Yoga-bhāṣya ascribed to Vyāsa who may or may not have accurately rendered the original sense, very probably moulding it to his own views."

Prof. Keith's remarks are not completely out of place. The text looks somewhat confused if it is interpreted solely with the aid of the traditional commentators, headed by Vyāsa. His Yoga-bhāṣya is the oldest and the most important commentary on the Yoga-Sutras. This, in turn, has several sub-commentaries — the earliest one known as the Tattva-Vaiśāradī by Vācaspati Miśra.

The flaw with these commentaries and sub-commentaries is that these were written at a time when the Pali Canon, containing the original teaching of the Buddha, had completely disappeared from India. The actual practice of insight-meditation taught by the Buddha had also disappeared. While Patanjali, the author of the Yoga-Sutras, could draw upon the oral as well as the living tradition of the Buddha's teaching, which were extant in his time, his commentators and sub-commentators remained ignorant of both. This fact itself seems to have resulted in inadequate—and, at times, uncalled for[3]—interpretations being offered by these commentators while explaining the Yoga-Sutras. The flaw can be rectified by

---

1. e.g., his aphorism on success in concentration through 'devotion to Lord' (*Samādhisiddhirīśvarapraṇidhānāt.* समाधिसिद्धिरीश्वरप्रणिधानात्। Y.S. II. 45).
2. 'A History of Sanskrit Literature' (Reprint 1948) (p. 490)
3. Even Tattva-Vaiśāradī, at times, finds fault with the Yoga-bhāṣya stating that it falls outside the scope of the sūtra. (Refer sub-comment on Y.S. IV. 15).

attempting a re-appraisal of the Yoga-Sutras in the light of the Buddha's teaching as enshrined in the Pali Canon.

It goes to Patanjali's credit that he was able to compile a systematic treatise on Yoga with just 194 aphorisms, using no more than 677 words. Obviously, the intrinsic worth of such a compact treatise can only be appreciated with the aid of detailed expositions which may throw light on the various topics as they come up for interpretation. This purpose is amply served by the Buddha's expositions which are quite elaborate.

There are several advantages of referring to the Buddha's expositions while interpreting the Yoga-Sutras: it brings one nearer to Patanjali's real point of view so far as most of his aphorisms are concerned; history of origin or detailed explanations of technical terms become available; the 'how' and 'why' of many aphorisms become clear; a large number of illustrations based on actual experience become handy; and one comes across a wealth of information having direct or indirect connection with any topic under consideration.

Examples of the above ad seriatim are:

- The aphorism "*Viśeṣadarśina ātmabhāvabhāvanāvinivṛttiḥ*"[1] ("विशेषदर्शिन आत्मभावभावनाविनिवृत्तिः") can be interpreted properly by assigning the meaning of "Vipassanā meditator" to the term *viśeṣa-darśī*" (विशेषदर्शी), taking this as the expanded form of "*vi-darśī*" (विदर्शी), Pali form "*vi-passī*" (विपस्सी).

- The origin of the term "*dharmamegha*" (धर्ममेघ)[2], the highest samādhi according to the Yoga-Sutras, can be traced to the word "*dhammamegha*" (धम्ममेघ) occurring in one of the Pali texts.[3]

---

1. Y.S. IV. 25
2. Y.S. IV. 29
3. Buddha-apadāna (बुद्ध-अपदान)

- The manner of diffusing loving-kindness, compassion, sympathetic joy and equanimity (*maitrī, karuṇā, muditā, upekṣā*) (मैत्री, करुणा, मुदिता, उपेक्षा) stands explained in the Buddha's teaching in detail,[1] while no such attempt has been made in the Yoga-bhāṣya while it explains the relevant aphorism.[2]

- One comes across several living examples substantiating the practice known as "*satyakriyā*" (सत्यक्रिया), Pali "*saccakiriyā*." (सच्चकिरिया). In this a truthful asseveration is made of acts done by the declarant, and by the power of this merit, the effect intended to be produced takes place, however amazing its character might be. No live examples have been cited in the Yoga-bhāṣya.[3]

One becomes knowledgeable about a number of disciples of the Buddha who possessed super-normal powers in an exceptional degree, e.g., *Sāriputta, Mahāmoggallāna, Anuruddha, Uppalavaṇṇā* (सारिपुत्त, महामोग्गल्लान, अनुरुद्ध, उप्पलवण्णा) and so on.[4] The Yoga-bhāṣya hardly cites any name.

The present work is only a small step in the direction of re-appraisal. The treatment of various matters in this book is by no means exhaustive. Much research is needed before all facts having a bearing on the subject can come to light.

Patanjali's Yoga-Sutras have been appended for purposes of ready reference.

We welcome constructive criticism of the book and invite suggestions for future.

Director,
Vipassana Research Institute,
Igatpuri

---

1. Majjhima. Mūla-paṇṇāsakaṃ (मज्झिम०, मूलपण्णासकं)- 7.4.8
2. Y.S. I. 33
3. Refer Y.S. II. 36
4. *Aṅguttara.* अङ्गुत्तर – 1.14.3

MODE OF TRANSLITERATION

OF
DEVANĀGARĪ INTO ROMAN SCRIPT

अ	आ	इ	ई	उ	ऊ	ए
a	ā	i	ī	u	ū	e
ऐ	ओ	औ	अं	अः	ऋ	
ai	o	au	ṃ	aḥ	ṛ	

क्	ख्	ग्	घ्	ङ्
k	kh	g	gh	ṅ
च्	छ्	ज्	झ्	ञ्
c	ch	j	jh	ñ
ट्	ठ्	ड्	ढ्	ण्
ṭ	ṭh	ḍ	ḍh	ṇ
त्	थ्	द्	ध्	न्
t	th	d	dh	n
प्	फ्	ब्	भ्	म्
p	ph	b	bh	m
य्	र्	ल्	व्	
y	r	l	v	
श्	ष्	स्	ह्	
ś	ṣ	s	h	
ळ्				
ḷ				

[N.B.]—Exceptions to this are words like पालि (*Pali*), पतञ्जलि (*Patanjali*), योगी (*Yogi*), योग-सूत्र (*Yoga-Sutras*), etc. Also the titles of books and names of authors listed under BIBLIOGRAPHY have been made to conform to their actual description on the books themselves.

ABBREVIATIONS

Aṅguttara (अङ्गुत्तर०)	- Aṅguttara-nikāya (अङ्गुत्तर-निकाय)
Cariyā (चरिया०)	- Cariyā-piṭaka (चरिया-पिटक)
Dīgha (दीघ०)	- Dīgha-nikāya (दीघ-निकाय)
Khuddaka (खुद्दक०)	- Khuddaka-pāṭha (खुद्दक-पाठ)
Majjhima (मज्झिम०)	- Majjhima-nikāya (मज्झिम-निकाय)
Paṭisambhidā (पटिसम्भिदा०)	- Paṭisambhidāmagga (पटिसम्भिदामग्ग)
Puggala (पुग्गल०)	- Puggala-paññatti (पुग्गल-पञ्ञत्ति)
Saṃyutta (संयुत्त०)	- Saṃyutta-nikāya (संयुत्त-निकाय)
Vinaya (विनय०)	- Vinaya-piṭaka (विनय-पिटक)
Visuddhi (विसुद्धि०)	- Visuddhimagga (विसुद्धिमग्ग)
Y.B.	- Yoga-bhāṣya
Y.S.	- Yoga-Sutras

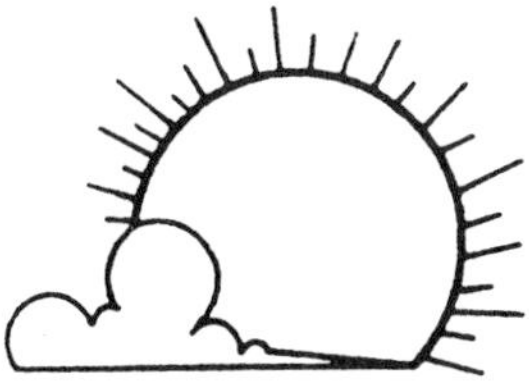

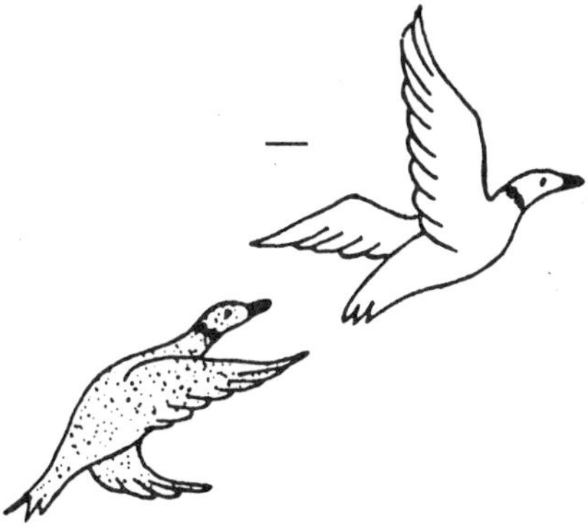

SECTION – I

MATTERS CONSISTENT WITH THE BUDDHA'S TEACHING

A. CONCEPTUAL

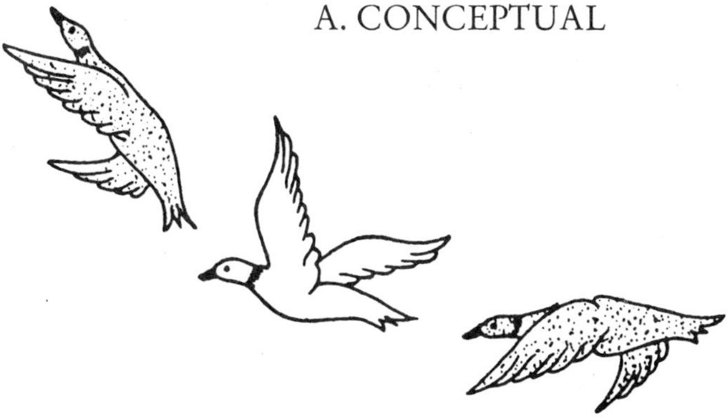

• Three aspects of suffering –

Patanjali speaks of three aspects of suffering, viz. *Pariṇāma-duḥkha* (परिणामदु:ख) (suffering due to mutation), *tāpa-duḥkha* (तापदु:ख) (suffering due to agony) and *saṃskāra-duḥkha* (संस्कारदु:ख) (suffering due to subliminal impressions).[1]

The Buddha also spoke of three states of suffering, viz. *dukkha-dukkhatā* (दुक्खदुक्खता), *saṅkhāra-dukkhatā* (सङ्खारदुक्खता) and *vipariṇāma-dukkhatā* (विपरिणामदुक्खता).[2]

The Buddha's *dukkha-dukkhatā* (दुक्खदुक्खता) and Patanjali's *tāpa-duḥkha* (तापदु:ख) have the same connotation since the terms *duḥkha* (दु:ख) and *tāpa* (ताप) are synonymous in the Sanskrit literature.

• To the discriminant there is nothing but suffering–

Patanjali asserts that for the discriminant there is nothing but suffering (*duḥkha*) (दु:ख) in this world.[3]

This forms the cardinal teaching of the Buddha also. According to him, there is suffering everywhere, even in joy, because there is always the anxiety of losing it and fear of what may happen when the pleasure has faded. When one discerns with discriminating knowledge, one finds that all formations

---

1. *Pariṇāma-tāpa-saṃskāra-duḥkhairguṇavṛtti-virodhācca duḥkhameva sarvaṃ vivekinaḥ.* (परिणाम-ताप-संस्कार-दु:खैर्गुणवृत्तिविरोधाच्च दु:खमेव सर्वं विवेकिन: ॥) (Y.S. II. 15)
2. "*Tisso imā, bhikkhave, dukkhatā. Katamā tisso? Dukkhadukkhatā, saṅkhāradukkhatā, vipariṇāma-dukkhatā—imā kho, bhikkhave, tisso dukkhatā . . .* " ("तिस्सो इमा, भिक्खवे, दुक्खता। कतमा तिस्सो ? दुक्ख-दुक्खता, सङ्खारदुक्खता, विपरिणामदुक्खता - इमा खो, भिक्खवे, तिस्सो दुक्खता।....") (*Saṃyutta* संयुत्त० – 45.165.167)
3. *Duḥkhameva sarvaṃ vivekinaḥ.* (दु:खमेव सर्वं विवेकिन: ०) (Y.S. II. 15)

whatsoever are nothing but suffering.[1] He also says what others call as 'pleasure' (*sukha*) (सुख), the Noble Ones acclaim as 'suffering' (*dukkha*) (दुक्ख).[2]

As a matter of fact, according to the Buddha, whatever sensations one experiences, all are nothing but suffering—that is to say, not only is *dukkha-vedanā* (दुक्ख-वेदना) (unpleasant sensation) a suffering, but *sukha-vedanā* (सुख-वेदना) (pleasant sensation) and *adukkhamasukha-vedanā* (अदुक्खमसुख-वेदना) (neutral sensation) are also suffering, because of their impermanent nature.[3]

Both the Buddha and Patanjali have the same expression to signify the aspect of pleasant feelings turning into 'suffering' as a result of change taking place—the Buddha calls it '*vipariṇāmadukkhatā*' ('विपरिणामदुक्खता')[4] and Patanjali '*pariṇāma-duḥkha*' ('परिणामदुःख')[5].

• 'Ignorance', as opposed to aspects of 'Wisdom' –

In the Yoga-Sutras the term *avidyā* (अविद्या) (Ignorance) has been defined as the (wrong) cognition of the eternal, the pure, the pleasant and the self in the non-eternal (*anitya*) (अनित्य), the impure (*aśuci*) (अशुचि), the painful (*duḥkha*) (दुःख) and the not-self (*anātma*) (अनात्म), respectively.[6]

---

1. '*Sabbe saṅkhārā dukkhā ti yadā paññāya passati*' ('सब्बे सङ्खारा दुक्खा ति यदा पञ्ञाय पस्सति।') (Thera-gāthā, थेरगाथा - 15.1.677)
2. '*Yaṃ pare sukhato āhu, tadariyā āhu dukkhato*' ('यं परे सुखतो आहु, तदरिया आहु दुक्खतो।') (Sutta-nipāta, सुत्तनिपात 3.12.361)
3. '*Yaṃ kiñci vedayitaṃ taṃ dukkhasmiṃ*' ('यं किञ्चि वेदयितं तं दुक्खस्मिं।') (Majjhima. Upari-paṇṇāsakaṃ (मज्झिम.। उपरिपण्णासकं।) (36.1.1.2)
4. *Saṃyutta* (संयुत्त०) 45.165.167
5. *Pariṇāma-tāpa-saṃskāra-duḥkhaiḥ.* (परिणाम-ताप-संस्कार-दुःखैः०) (Y.S. II. 15)
6. *Anityāśuciduḥkhānātmasu nityaśucisukhātmakhyātiravidyā.* (अनित्याशुचिदुःखानात्मसु नित्यशुचिसुखात्मख्यातिरविद्या) (Y.S. II. 5)

The above definition reminds one of the aspects of wisdom known as *anicca* (अनिच्च), *anattā* (अनत्ता), *dukkha* (दुक्ख) and *asubha* (असुभ) (that is, non-eternal, not-self, pain and impure) in the Buddha's teaching.[1]

• The four sublime states –

The serenity of mind has been stated to arise from the inculcation of loving-kindness (*maitrī*) (मैत्री), compassion (*karuṇā*) (करुणा), altruistic joy (*muditā*) (मुदिता) and nonchalance (*upekṣā*) (उपेक्षा) towards happiness and sorrow, merit and demerit, respectively.[2]

These four qualities mentioned in the Yoga-Sutras are just the four states called *appamañña* (अप्पमञ्ञ) (Boundless States) or *'brahmavihāra-s'* (ब्रह्मविहार) (Sublime Abodes) in the Buddha's teaching. These are named as *mettā* (मेत्ता), *karuṇā* (करुणा), *muditā* (मुदिता) and *upekkhā* (उपेक्खा) in exactly the same order.[3]

• Four types of 'Karma' –

It has been asserted that a yogi's 'Karma' is neither-white-nor-black (*aśuklākṛṣṇaṃ*) (अशुक्लाकृष्णं) while the 'Karma' of others is of three kinds (*trividham*) (त्रिविधम्)[4]. Thus, in all, four types of 'Karmas' have been referred to.

This is what the Buddha had also, precisely, taught, naming the 'Karmas' (*kamma*) (कम्म) as black (*kaṇha*) (कण्ह),

---

1. *Anicce niccasaññino, dukkhe ca sukhasaññino, anattani ca attā ti, asubhe subhasaññino.* (अनिच्चे निच्चसञ्ञिनो, दुक्खे च सुखसञ्ञिनो, अनत्तनि च अत्ता ति, असुभे सुभसञ्ञिनो।) (*Paṭisambhidā.* पटिसम्भिदा. 1.8.2.3)
2. *Maitrīkaruṇāmuditopekṣāṇāṃ sukhaduḥkhapuṇyāpuṇyaviśayāṇāṃ bhāvanātaścittaprasādanam.* (मैत्रीकरुणामुदितोपेक्षाणां सुखदुःखपुण्यापुण्यविषयाणां भावनातश्चित्तप्रसादनम्॥) (Y.S. I.33)
3. *Vibhaṅga (विभङ्ग)* (13.1.13)
4. *Karmāśuklākṛṣṇaṃ yoginastrividhamitareṣām.* (कर्माशुक्लाकृष्णं योगिनस्त्रिविधमितरेषाम्॥) (Y.S. IV. 7)

white (*sukka*) (सुक्क), black-and-white (*kaṇhasukka*) (कण्हसुक्क) and neither black-nor-white (*akaṇha asukka*) (अकण्ह असुक्क).[1]

• The four divisions of Yoga –

There are four divisions of Yoga (*yogavyūha*) (योगव्यूह), viz., the suffering, its cause, its cessation and the means of cessation. These have been termed *heya* (हेय), *heyahetu* (हेयहेतु), *hāna* (हान) and *hānopāya* (हानोपाय), respectively.[2]

This division follows the pattern of the Four Noble Truths (*ariya-sacca*) (अरिय-सच्च) enunciated by the Buddha. These are: the truth of suffering, the truth of the origin of suffering, the truth of the cessation of suffering, and the truth of the Noble Eightfold Path leading to the cessation of suffering. The terms used for these are: *dukkha* (दुक्ख), *dukkha-samudaya* (दुक्खसमुदय), *dukkha-nirodha* (दुक्खनिरोध) and *dukkhanirodha-gāminī paṭipadā* (दुक्खनिरोधगामिनी पटिपदा).

Parallel to the expression *hāna* (हान) used by Patanjali, the word frequently met with in the Buddha's teaching is *pahāna* (पहान), e.g., *pahānaṃ kāmasaññānaṃ* (पहानं कामसञ्ञानं)[3], while the word *hāna* (हान) is used as a part of compound words, e.g., *hānabhāgiyā saññā* (हानभागिया सञ्ञा).[4]

• Abstentions: the first limb of the Yoga –

The first of the eight limbs of Yoga is called *yamāḥ* (यमाः) (Abstentions). These comprise abstention from injury (*ahiṃsā*) (अहिंसा), falsehood (*satya*) (सत्य), theft (*asteya*) (अस्तेय), incontinence (*abrahmacarya*) (अब्रह्मचर्य) and possessing

---

1. *Kammaṃ kaṇhaṃ . . . sukkaṃ . . . kaṇhasukkaṃ . . . akaṇhaṃ asukkaṃ.* (कम्मं कण्हं....सुक्कं....कण्हसुक्कं...अकण्हं असुक्कं.... ।) (Aṅguttara. अङ्गुत्तर० – 4.24.2.1)
2. Y.S. (II. 16,17,25,26)
3. *Aṅguttara.* (अङ्गुत्तर०) 3.4.3.
4. *Aṅguttara.* (अङ्गुत्तर०) 4.18.9

things (*aparigraha*) (अपरिग्रह).[1]

Three divisions of the Noble Eight-fold Path discovered by the Buddha known as *sammā-kammanto* (सम्मा-कम्मन्तो), *sammā-vācā* (सम्मा-वाचा) and *sammā-saṅkappo* (सम्मा-सङ्कप्पो) (i.e., Right Bodily Action, Right Speech and Right Thought) recommend all the above and a few more.[2]

- **Factors helping the attainment of Cessation (*Nirodha*) (निरोध) –**

According to the Yoga-Sutras, the factors which help the attainment of 'nirodha' by ordinary yogis are *śraddhā* (श्रद्धा) (Faith), *vīrya* (वीर्य) (Energy), *smṛti* (स्मृति) (Mindfulness), *samādhi* (समाधि) (Concentration of the Mind) and *prajñā* (प्रज्ञा) (Intuitive Knowledge).[3]

According to the Buddha, the self-same factors, viz. *saddhā* (सद्धा), *viriya* (विरिय), *sati* (सति), *samādhi* (समाधि) and *paññā* (पञ्ञा) constitute the five mental strengths (*bala-s*) (बल).[4] These are also called five faculties (indriya-s) (इन्द्रिय)[5] on the consideration that when one starts mastering

1. *Tatrāhiṃsāsatyāsteyabrahmacaryāparigrahā yamāḥ.* (तत्राहिंसासत्यास्तेयब्रह्मचर्यापरिग्रहा यमाः ॥) (Y.S. II.30)
2. *Pāṇātipātā veramaṇī (i.e., ahiṃsā), musāvādā veramaṇī (i.e., satya), adinnādānā veramaṇī (i.e., asteya), kāmesu micchācārā veramaṇī (i.e., brahmacarya), nekkhamma saṅkappo (i.e., aparigraha), (Vibhaṅga-4.1.9).* (पाणातिपाता वेरमणी (अहिंसा), मुसावादा वेरमणी (सत्य), अदिन्नादाना वेरमणी (अस्तेय), कामेसु मिच्छाचारा वेरमणी (ब्रह्मचर्य), नेक्खम्म सङ्कप्पो (अपरिग्रह) (विभङ्ग 4.1.9)
3. *Śraddhāvīryasmṛtisamādhiprajñāpūrvaka itareṣām.* (श्रद्धावीर्यस्मृतिसमाधिप्रज्ञापूर्वक इतरेषाम् ॥) (Y.S. I.20)
4. *"Pañcimāni, bhikkhave, balāni. Katamāni pañca? Saddhābalaṃ, viriyabalaṃ, satibalaṃ, samādhibalaṃ, paññābalaṃ - imāni kho, bhikkhave, pañca balānī" ti.* (पञ्चिमानि, भिक्खवे, बलानि। कतमानि पञ्च? सद्धाबलं, विरियबलं, सतिबलं, समाधिबलं, पञ्ञाबलं - इमानि खो, भिक्खवे, पञ्च बलानी" ति।) (Aṅguttara. अङ्गुत्तर० - 5.21.4)
5. *Pañcindriyāni: saddhindriyaṃ, viriyindriyaṃ, satindriyaṃ, samādhindriyaṃ, paññidriyaṃ.* (पञ्चिन्द्रियानि: सद्धिन्द्रियं, विरियिन्द्रियं,

them, they begin to help in attaining the final goal of full liberation.

• Three kinds of Intuitive Knowledge (*Prajñā*) (**प्रज्ञा**) –

According to Patanjali, when confidence develops in concentration without sustained attention to the object of meditation (*nirvicāra samādhi*) (निर्विचार समाधि), there arises inner quietude.[1] In that state there arises the truth-bearing Intuitive Knowledge (*ṛtambharā prajñā*) (ऋतम्भरा प्रज्ञा).[2] This Intuitive Knowledge stands on a different footing from the two other kinds of intuitive knowledge (*prajñā*) (प्रज्ञा)—which go by the names of *śruta* (श्रुत) (what is heard) and *anumāna* (what is inferred)—the reason being that it has a different purpose and has a special significance (*viśeṣārthatvāt*) (विशेषार्थत्वात्).[3]

The Buddha had also dwelt upon three kinds of Intuitive Knowledge (*paññā*) (पञ्ञा): *sutamayā* (सुतमया) (received), *cintanamayā* (चिन्तनमया) (intellectual) and *bhāvanāmayā* (भावनामया) (experiential).[4] Out of these it is the last one that purifies the mind and is, therefore, significantly different from the other two.

Since the *bhāvanāmayā paññā* (भावनामया पञ्ञा) is based on one's own experience and is totally free from the elements of imagination or speculation, it reveals the inherent truth. Thus,

---

सतिन्द्रियं, समाधिन्द्रियं, पञ्ञिन्द्रियं। (Dīgha. Pāthikavaggo दीघ.। पाथिकवग्गो। 11.1.6)

1. *Nirvicāravaiśāradye'dhyātmaprasādaḥ.* (निर्विचारवैशारद्येऽध्यात्मप्रसादः ॥) (Y.S. I.47)
2. *Ṛtambharā tatra prajñā.* (ऋतम्भरा तत्र प्रज्ञा ॥) (Y.S. I.48)
3. *Śrutānumānaprajñābhyāmanyaviśayā viśeṣārthatvāt.* (श्रुतानुमानप्रज्ञाभ्यामन्यविषया विशेषार्थत्वात् ॥) (Y.S. I.49)
4. *Sutamayā (parato sutvā paṭilabhati), cintanamayā (parato assutvā paṭilabhati, bhāvanāmayā (sabbāpi samāpannassa paññā).* सुतमया (परतो सुत्वा पटिलभति) | चिन्तनमया (परतो अस्सुत्वा पटिलभति) | भावनामया (सब्बापि समापन्नस्स पञ्ञा) | (Vibhaṅga. विभङ्ग – 16.2.29).

the *ṛtambharā prajñā* (ऋतम्भरा प्रज्ञा)[1] of Patanjali has to be taken in the sense of *bhāvanāmayā paññā* (भावनामया पञ्ञा) as enunciated by the Buddha.

For the Buddha, *ṛta* (ऋत) (Truth) was Law of Nature, which he expressed as *dhammaṭṭhitatā* (धम्मट्ठितता) or *dhamma-niyāmatā* (धम्मनियामता). He explained that the Law of Nature exists irrespective of the fact whether a Fully Enlightened Person exists or not.[2] All that a Fully Enlightened Person does is to gain a perfect insight into this law and then reveal it to others.[3]

• The set of mental defilements –

The Yoga of Action (*kriyāyoga*) (क्रियायोग) is stated to have for its purpose the development of *samādhi* (समाधि) and the attenuation of mental defilements (*kleśa-s*) (क्लेश). These defilements have been spelt out as *avidyā* (अविद्या) (Ignorance), *asmitā* (अस्मिता) (Egoism), *rāga* (राग) (Craving), *dveṣa* (द्वेष) (Aversion) and *abhiniveśa* (अभिनिवेश) (Clinging to one's own life).[4]

The Buddha named ten defilements (*kilesa-s*) (किलेस), viz. *lobha* (लोभ) (Greed), *dosa* (दोस) (Aversion), *moha* (मोह) (Delusion), *māna* (मान) (Conceit), *diṭṭhi* (दिट्ठि) (Speculative Views), *vicikicchā* (विचिकिच्छा) (Sceptical Doubt), *thina* (थिन) (Mental Torpor), *uddhacca* (उद्धच्च) (Restlessness), *ahirika*

---

1. Y.S. (I. 48)
2. *Uppādā vā, bhikkhave, tathāgatānaṃ anuppādā vā tathāgatānaṃ, thitā va sā dhātu dhammaṭṭhitatā dhammaniyāmatā.* (उप्पादा वा, भिक्खवे, तथागतानं अनुप्पादा वा तथागतानं, ठिता व सा धातु धम्मट्ठितता धम्मनियामता) (Aṅguttara. अङ्गुत्तर॰ – 3.14.4)
3. *Abhisambujjhitvā abhisametvā ācikkhati deseti paññāpeti paṭṭhapeti vivarati.* (अभिसम्बुज्झित्वा अभिसमेत्वा आचिक्खति देसेति पञ्ञापेति पट्ठपेति विवरति) (Aṅguttara. अङ्गुत्तर॰ – 3.14.4)
4. *Avidyāsmitārāgadveṣābhiniveśāḥ.* (अविद्यास्मितारागद्वेषाभिनिवेशाः ॥) (Y.S. II.3)

(अहिरिक) (Shamelessness) and *anottappa* (अनोत्तप्प) (Unconscientiousness).[1] Out of these, Patanjali seems to have picked up the first four as *lobha* (लोभ) corresponds to *rāga* (राग) and *abhiniveśa* (अभिनिवेश), *dosa* (दोस) to *dveṣa* (द्वेष), *moha* (मोह) to *avijjā* (अविज्जा) and *māna* (मान) to *asmitā* (अस्मिता).

• The Characteristics of the 'Lord' (*Īśvara*) (ईश्वर) –

According to the Yoga-Sutras, the 'Lord' (*Īśvara*) (ईश्वर) is a special kind of Person (*puruśaviśeṣah*) (पुरुषविशेषः), unaffected by hindrances (*kleśa*) (क्लेश), actions (*karma*) (कर्म), results (*vipāka*) (विपाक) and latent-deposits (*āśaya*) (आशय).[2]

In the Buddha's terminology, such a person would be called an *arahant* (अर्हन्त्) since he, too, remains unaffected by hindrances (*kilesa*) (किलेस), actions (*kamma*) (कम्म), results (*vipāka*) (विपाक) and latent-deposits (*āsaya*) (आसय).

It is worth noting that Patanjali, like the Buddha, does not envisage any 'Lord' (*Īśvara*) (ईश्वर) exercising control over worldly phenomena, including human action. Both lay stress not on the 'power' but 'purity' aspect of *Īśvara* (ईश्वर) (the 'Lord').

• Definitions of 'Craving' and 'Aversion' –

In the Yoga-Sutras the terms *rāga* (राग) (Craving) and *dveṣa* (द्वेष) (Aversion) have been defined as experiences with latent-bias (*anuśayī*) (अनुशयी) of pleasure and pain, respectively.[3]

The use of the word *anuśayī* (अनुशयी) (i.e., with latent-bias) above suggests the influence of the Buddha's

---

1. These are explained in the *Dhammasaṅgaṇi* (धम्मसङ्गणि) – 3.1.97 and enumerated in *Vibhaṅga* (विभङ्ग) – 17.11.199.
2. *Kleśakarmavipākāśayairaparāmṛṣṭaḥ puruṣaviśeṣa Īśvaraḥ.* (क्लेशकर्मविपाकाशयैरपरामृष्टः पुरुषविशेष ईश्वरः ॥) (Y.S. I.24)
3. *Sukhānuśayī rāgaḥ. Duḥkhānuśayī dveṣaḥ.* (सुखानुशयी रागः ॥ दुःखानुशयी द्वेषः ॥) (Y.S. II. 7-8)

teaching which, too, speaks of latent-biases, such as *kāmarāgānusayo* (कामरागानुसयो) (latent-bias for Sensuous Greed), *paṭighānusayo* (पटिघानुसयो) (latent-bias for Repugnance) and so on.[1] The latent-bias for Sensuous Greed is in the nature of Craving (*rāga*) (राग) and the one for Repugnance is in the nature of Aversion (*dveṣa*) (द्वेष).

The Buddha is known to have destroyed his latent-biases (*anusaya-s*) (अनुसय)[2].

- **Saṃvega (संवेग) as a stirring force for emancipation –**

It has been stated that for those who apply themselves to the task with great fervour (*saṃvega*) (संवेग), the *nirodha* (निरोध) (cessation) is near at hand.[3]

The Buddha's teaching is full of references where, on fervour (*saṃvega*) (संवेग) being induced, the person concerned attained the state of full liberation not long thereafter.[4]

The Buddha was a staunch advocate of *saṃvega* (संवेग).[5]

- **Thought-conceptions (*vitarka-s*) (वितर्क) and their three aspects –**

In the Yoga-Sutras thought-conceptions (*vitarkāḥ*) (वितर्का:), such as injury, etc. (*hiṃsādayaḥ*) (हिंसादय:) have been

---

1. *Aṅguttara.* (अङ्गुत्तर०) – 7.2.1
2. *Tuvaṃ buddho tuvaṃ satthā, tuvaṃ mārābhibhū muni. Tuvaṃ anusaye chetvā, tiṇṇo tārasimaṃ pajaṃ.* (तुवं बुद्धो तुवं सत्था, तुवं माराभिभू मुनि। तुवं अनुसये छेत्वा, तिण्णो तारसिमं पजं॥) *(Majjhima. Majjhima-paṇṇāsakaṃ.* मज्झिम० मज्झिम-पण्णासकं – 42.4.6)
3. *Tīvrasaṃvegānāmāsannaḥ.* (तीव्रसंवेगानामासन्न: ॥) (Y.S. I.21)
4. *E.g., etamādīnavaṃ ñatvā, saṃvegaṃ alabhiṃ tadā. Mohaṃ viddho tadā santo, sampatto āsavakkhayaṃ.* (एतमादीनवं ञत्वा, संवेगं अलभिं तदा। मोहं विद्धो तदा सन्तो, सम्पत्तो आसवक्खयं॥) *(Theragāthā.* थेरगाथा – 16.4.791) *For more references see Thera-gāthā* (थेरगाथा) (6.1.375-380 and 8.3.510-517)
5. *Ātāpino saṃvegino bhavātha.* (आतापिनो संवेगिनो भवाथ।) (Dhammapada, धम्मपद – 10.144)

shown to have three aspects—done, caused to be done or approved.[1]

The Buddha referred to these very aspects when he said:

"Monks, one possessed of three qualities is put into Hell according to his deserts. What three?

"One is himself a taker of life, encourages another to do the same, and approves thereof."[2]

Patanjali has not named the various types of thought-conceptions and has merely referred to them as *vitarkā hiṃsādayaḥ* (वितर्का हिंसादय:) (i.e., thought-conceptions such as injury, etc.). These have, however, been amplified in the Buddha's teaching as *vihiṃsā* (विहिंसा), *vyāpāda* (व्यापाद), *kāma* (काम) (injury, malevolence, sensuality) and *a-vihiṃsā* (अ-विहिंसा), *a-vyāpāda* (अ-व्यापाद) and *nekkhamma* (नेक्खम्म), as their opposites. Out of these the first three are karmically un-wholesome and the last three otherwise.

In the Buddha's exposition the term *vitakka* (वितक्क) (Skt. *Vitarka*) (वितर्क) has two meanings: 1. Contact of an object with any of the six sense-doors, and 2. thought-conception.

• Oppression by a thought-conception (*vitarka*) (वितर्क): the way to get rid of –

In the Yoga-Sutras it has been prescribed that, if one feels oppressed by a thought-conception, one may reflect on the

1. *Vitarkā hiṃsādayaḥ kṛtakāritānumoditāḥ.* (वितर्का हिंसादय: कृतकारितानुमोदिता:० ॥) (Y.S. II.34)
2. *"Tīhi, bhikkhave, dhammehi samannāgato yathābhataṃ nikkhitto evaṃ niraye. Katemehi tīhi? Attanā ca pāṇātipātī hoti, parañca pāṇātipāte samādapeti, pāṇātipāte ca samanuñño hoti."* ("तीहि, भिक्खवे, धम्मेहि समन्नागतो यथाभतं निक्खित्तो एवं निरये। कतमेहि तीहि? अत्तना च पाणातिपाती होति, परं च पाणातिपाते समादपेति, पाणातिपाते च समनुञ्ञो होति।") (Aṅguttara. अङ्गुत्तर० – 3.17.1)

opposite one.[1]

This prescription is in consonance with the Buddha's teaching which lays down reflection on contrary thoughts in the following manner:

(a) reflection on loathsomeness to overcome craving;

(b) reflection on loving-kindness to overcome aversion; and

(c) reflection on inner wisdom to overcome delusion.[2]

- **Powers connected with the sublime states –**

The Yoga-Sutras speak of powers (*balāni*) (बलानि) flowing from constraint upon Loving-kindness (*maitrī*) (मैत्री) and other sublime states.[3]

According to the Buddha's teaching, several benefits accrue to one who is given to *mettābhāvanā* (मेत्ताभावना) (Loving-kindness). These are: one sleeps in comfort, wakes in comfort, dreams no evil dreams, is dear to human beings, is dear to non-human beings, is guarded by deities, remains un-affected by fire, poison and weapons and, though one may penetrate not the beyond, one reaches the Brahmā World.[4]

---

1. *Vitarkabādhane pratipakṣabhāvanaṃ.* (वितर्कबाधने प्रतिपक्षभावनम् ॥) (Y.S. II. 33)
2. *Rāgassa pahānāya asubhā bhāvetabbā, dosassa pahānāya mettā bhāvetabbā, mohassa pahānāya paññā bhāvetabbā.* (रागस्स पहानाय असुभा भावेतब्बा, दोसस्स पहानाय मेत्ता भावेतब्बा, मोहस्स पहानाय पञ्ञा भावेतब्बा।) (Aṅguttara. अङ्गुत्तर॰ – 6.11.1)
3. *Maitryādiṣu balāni.* (मैत्र्यादिषु बलानि ॥) (Y.S. III. 22)
4. *"Sukhaṃ supati, sukhaṃ paṭibujjhati, na pāpakaṃ supinaṃ passati, manussānaṃ piyo hoti, a-manussānaṃ piyo hoti, devatā rakkhanti, nāssa aggi vā visaṃ vā satthaṃ vā kamati, uttari appaṭivijjhanto brahmalokūpago hoti."* ("सुखं सुपति, सुखं पटिबुज्झति, न पापकं सुपिनं पस्सति, मनुस्सानं पियो होति, अमनुस्सानं पियो होति, देवता रक्खन्ति, नास्स अग्गि वा विसं वा सत्थं वा कमति, उत्तरि अप्पटिविज्झन्तो ब्रह्मलोकूपगो होति।") (Aṅguttara. अङ्गुत्तर॰ 8.1.1)

• Suspension of enmity in the presence of one firmly established in Abstinence from Injury –

The Yoga-Sutras state when one is firmly established in abstinence from injury (*ahiṃsā*) (अहिंसा), one's presence begets a suspension of enmity (*vairatyāgaḥ*) (वैरत्यागः).[1]

The Pali Canon abounds in such assertions: for instance, "One whose mind is given to non-injury to others all the time develops amity for all. Nobody harbours enmity against him."[2]

It is also common knowledge that the furious elephant Nāḷāgiri became calm and quiet in the presence of the Buddha, who was firmly established in Abstinence from Injury and was, for that matter, an Apostle of Non-violence and always radiating Loving-kindness (*mettā*) (मेत्ता). Loving-kindness has a wonderful effect not only on human beings but also on animals.[3]

There is, however, a curious reference in the *Pañcatantra* (पञ्चतन्त्र) that the great grammarian Paṇini (पाणिनि) was killed by a lion, the sage Jaimini (जैमिनि) by an elephant and Piṅgalācārya (पिङ्गलाचार्य) by a crocodile.[4] Could it be that these

---

1. *Ahiṃsāpratiṣṭhāyāṃ tatsannidhau vairatyāgaḥ* . . . (अहिंसाप्रतिष्ठायां तत्सन्निधौ वैरत्यागः ॥) (Y.S. II.25)
2. "*Yassa sabbamahorattaṃ, ahiṃsāya rato mano; Mettaṃ so sabbabhūtesu, veraṃ tassa na kenacī" ti.* ("यस्स सब्बमहोरत्तं, अहिंसाय रतो मनो। मेत्तं सो सब्बभूतेसु, वेरं तस्स न केनची" ति) Saṃyutta 1/209 Maṇibhadda Sutta (संयुत्त १.२०९ मणिभद्द सुत्त ॥)
3. *Nāḷāgiriṃ gajavaraṃ atimattabhūtaṃ, dāvaggi cakkamasanīva sudāruṇantaṃ, mettambuseka vidhinā jitavā munindo, taṃ tejasā bhavatu te jayamaṅgalāni.* (नाळागिरिं गजवरं अतिमत्तभूतं, दावग्गि चक्कमसनीव सुदारुणन्तं। मेत्तम्बुसेक विधिना जितवा मुनिन्दो, तं तेजसा भवतु ते जयमङ्गलानि ॥) (*Jayamaṅgala-aṭṭhagāthā* (जयमङ्गलअट्ठगाथा - ३) For details of this incident, refer Vinaya, Cullavaggo (विनय. चुल्लवग्गो) – 7.8.13.
4. *Siṃho vyākaraṇasya karturaharat, prāṇānpriyānpāṇineḥ. Mīṃāṃsākṛtamunmamātha sahesā, hastī muniṃ Jaiminiṃ. Chandojñānanidhiṃ jaghāna makaro, velātaṭe Piṅgalaṃ. Ajñānāvṛtacetasāmatiruṣāṃ, ko'rthastiraścāṃ guṇaiḥ.*

celebrities who wrote wonderful treatises on *vyākaraṇa* (व्याकरण) (grammar), *mīmāṃsā* (मीमांसा) (one of the six chief systems of Indian philosophy) and *chhandaḥśāstra* (छन्द:शास्त्र) (prosody) did not know how to radiate Loving-kindness (*mettā*) (मेत्ता)?

• 'Contentment' as a source of highest happiness –

According to the Yoga-Sutras, from Contentment (*santoṣa*) (सन्तोष) one gets the highest happiness.[1]

According to the Pali Canon, Contentment (*santosa*) (सन्तोस) is wealth *par excellence.*[2] It is one of the three disciplines to be cultivated by a wise bhikkhu from the very beginning.[3]

• Subduing action (mastering power) of the mind –

After pointing out certain supports (*ālambana-s*) (आलम्बन) for concentration of the mind,[4] the Yoga-Sutras assert that the subduing action (*vaśīkāra*) (वशीकार) of the mind has for its limits extreme smallness and extreme greatness (*paramāṇuparamamahatvāntaḥ*) (परमाणुपरममहत्त्वान्त:).[5]

(सिंहो व्याकरणस्य कर्तुरहरत्, प्राणान्प्रियान्पाणिने:।
मीमांसाकृतमुन्ममाथ सहसा, हस्ती मुनिं जैमिनिम्॥
छन्दोज्ञाननिधिं जघान मकरो, वेलातटे पिङ्गलम्।
अज्ञानावृतचेतसामतिरुषां, कोऽर्थस्तिरश्चां गुणै:॥) (Pañcatantra, पञ्चतंत्र – 2.23)

1. *Santoṣādanuttamaḥ sukhalābhaḥ* (सन्तोषादनुत्तम: सुखलाभ:॥) (Y.S. II. 42)
2. *Santuṭṭhiparamaṃ dhanaṃ* (सन्तुट्ठिपरमं धनं) (Dhammapada, धम्मपद - 15.204)
3. *Tatrāyamādi bhavati, idha paññassa bhikkhuno; Indriyagutti santuṭṭhi, pātimokkhe ca saṃvaro.*
   (तत्रायमादि भवति, इध पञ्ञस्स भिक्खुनो।
   इन्द्रियगुत्ति सन्तुट्ठि, पातिमोक्खे च संवरो॥)
   (Dhammapada, धम्मपद – 25.375)
4. Y.S. (I.35 – 39)
5. *Paramāṇuparamamahatvānto'sya vaśīkāraḥ.* (परमाणुपरममहत्त्वान्तोऽस्य वशीकार:॥) (Y.S. I.40)

According to the Buddha's teaching also, by means of the *Earth-Kasiṇa* (पठवी-कसिण) (which is one of the forty supports for concentration of mind) one succeeds in reaching the stage of mastery with regard to small and boundless objects.[1]

• Blazing forth of light from the body –

From the conquest of *Samāna* (a vital air), a yogi is said to be surrounded by a blaze of light.[2]

A number of events refer to the effulgence of light from the Buddha's body. On two occasions, however, the skin of a Tathāgata is stated to become exceedingly bright: the night He attains perfect insight and the night He passes away finally.[3]

• Mind-like velocity –

According to the Yoga-Sutras, a yogi can command rapidity of physical movement—of the same order as that of the mind.[4]

The Buddha's lore refers to his crossing of the Ganges at Pāṭaligāma when the river was in spate. He is stated to have crossed it "as instantaneously as a strong man would stretch forth his arm and draw it back again", vanishing from one bank, re-appearing instantly on the opposite.[5]

• Mastery over actions and their consequences –

It has been asserted if a yogi establishes himself in Truthfulness (*satya*) (सत्य), this would result in his gaining mastery over actions and their consequences.[6]

---

1. *Visuddhi.* (विसुद्धि॰) (V. 28)
2. *Samānajayājjvalanaṃ* (समानजयाज्ज्वलनम् ॥) (Y.S. III. 40)
3. *Dīgha. Mahāvaggo* (दीघ॰ । महावग्गो ।) 3.21.68
4. *Tato manojavitvaṃ.* (ततो मनोजवित्वं॰ ॥) (Y.S. III 48)
5. *Dīgha. Mahāvaggo.* (दीघ॰ । महावग्गो ।) 3.6.24
6. *Satyapratiṣṭhāyāṃ kriyāphalāśrayatvam.* (सत्यप्रतिष्ठायां क्रियाफलाश्रयत्वम् ॥) (Y.S. II.36)

In Buddha's time this phenomenon was known as *saccakiriyā* (सच्चकिरिया) (Skt. *Satyakriyā*) (सत्यक्रिया). In this a truthful asseveration was made of acts done by the declarant either in this or some former birth, and by the power of this merit, the effect intended to be produced took place, however wonderful its character might have been. Two instances are cited below:

1) "Since the time I recollect myself and ever since I have become wise, I know for certain that I have not hurt even a single creature. With this truthful declaration of mine, may the Rain pour down!"[1]

2) "May Truth help me now in my assertion as It will in future also. I know for certain that there is no one dearer to me than you. With this truthful declaration of mine, may your ailment pass off!"[2]

• Knowledge of another's mind –

In the Yoga-Sutras it is mentioned that one can have knowledge of another's mind (*paracittajñānaṃ*) (परचित्तज्ञानं) through concentration on his notions (*pratyaya*) (प्रत्यय)[3]. But one would not know the support (or basis) of these notions.[4] The Yoga-bhāṣya illustrates this by stating that while such a

---

1. *"Yato sarāmi attānaṃ yato pattosmi viññutaṃ, nābhijānāmi sañcicca ekampāṇaṃ vihiṃsitaṃ. Etena saccavajjena pajjunno abhivassatu."*
(“यतो सरामि अत्तानं यतो पत्तोस्मि विञ्ञुतं,
नाभिजानामि सञ्चिच्च एकम्पाणं विहिंसितं।
एतेन सच्चवज्जेन पज्जुन्नो अभिवस्सतु) (Cariyā. चरिया. – 5.4.6)

2. *"Tathā maṃ saccaṃ pāletu pālayissati ce mamaṃ yathāhaṃ nābhijānāmi aññaṃ piyataraṃ tathā. Etena saccavajjena vyādhi te vūpasammatu."*
(“तथा मं सच्चं पालेतु पालयिस्सति चे ममं
यथाहं नाभिजानामि अञ्ञं पियतरं तथा।
एतेन सच्चवज्जेन व्याधि ते वूपसम्मतु॥) (Jātaka. जातक० – 519.27)

3. Pratyayasya paracittajñānaṃ (प्रत्ययस्य परचित्तज्ञानम्) (Y.S. III.14)

4. *Na ca tatsālambanaṃ tasyāviṣayībhūtatvāt.* (न च तत्सालम्बनं तस्या वेषयीभूतत्वात्॥) (Y.S. III. 20)

yogi would come to know that the other person is full of craving he would not know what might be its basis.

In the Buddha's teaching also, there is a super-normal knowledge called *ceto-pariya-ñāṇaṃ* (चेतो-परिय-ञाणं) (knowledge of another's mind). This knowledge also is attained through utmost perfection in mental concentration. Such a person "knows the minds of other beings by penetrating them with his own mind. He knows the greedy mind as greedy and the not-greedy as not greedy; and so on".[1] Thus, here also the practitioner does not know the basis of the mind's character at a given point of time although he would know its quality.

• Knowledge of previous existences through direct perception of the subliminal impressions (*saṃskāra-s*) (संस्कार) –

The Yoga-Sutras assert that knowledge of previous existences (*pūrvajātijñānaṃ*) (पूर्वजातिज्ञानं) accrues through direct perception of subliminal impressions (*saṃskārasākṣātkaraṇāt*) (संस्कारसाक्षात्करणात्).[2] Elsewhere, it has been stated that recollection (*smṛti*) (स्मृति) and subliminal impressions (*saṃskāra-s*) (संस्कार) have the same characteristic.[3] This implies that knowledge of previous existences would accrue through direct perception of recollections also.

This is what, precisely, the Buddha had taught –

---

1. *So parasattānaṃ parapuggalānaṃ cetasā ceto paricca pajānāti—sarāgaṃ vā cittaṃ sarāgaṃ cittaṃ ti pajānāti, vītarāgaṃ vā cittaṃ vītarāgaṃ cittaṃ ti pajānāti.* (सो परसत्तानं परपुग्गलानं चेतसा चेतो परिच्च पजानाति - सरागं वा चित्तं सरागं चित्तं ति पजानाति, वीतरागं वा चित्तं वीतरागं चित्तं ति पजानाति० ।) (Dīgha. Sīlakkhandhavaggo दीघ० । सीलक्खन्धवग्गो । 2.5.93)
2. *Saṃskārasākṣātkaraṇāt pūrvajātijñānam.* (संस्कारसाक्षात्करणात् पूर्वजातिज्ञानम् ॥) (Y.S. III. 18)
3. *Smṛtisaṃskārayorekarūpatvāt.* (स्मृतिसंस्कारयोरेकरूपत्वात् ॥) (Y.S. IV. 9)

"O bhikkhus, which phenomena are to be directly perceived? The previous existence, O bhikkus, should be directly perceived through recollection."[1]

• Knowledge of Death (*aparāntajñānam*) (अपरान्तज्ञानम्)–

According to the Yoga-Sutras, a yogi can acquire the knowledge of Death.[2]

The Buddha had himself forecast his Death: "At the end of three months from now, the Tathāgata will pass away."[3]

• Disappearing from view (*antardhānam*) (अन्तर्धानम्) –

According to the Yoga-Sutras, a yogi can attain the power of suddenly disappearing from view.[4]

A canonical text states that after the Buddha had given Dhamma discourses in Assemblies of Nobles in various spheres of the Universe he would vanish, while the congregation would keep wondering: "Who may this be that has thus vanished away—a man or a god?[5]

---

1. *"Katame ca, bhikkhave, dhammā satiyā sacchikaraṇīyā? Pubbenivāso, bhikkhave, satiyā sacchikaraṇīyo."* ("कतमे च, भिक्खवे, धम्मा सतिया सच्छिकरणीया? पुब्बेनिवासो, भिक्खवे, सतिया सच्छिकरणीयो।") (Aṅguttara. अङ्गुत्तर – 4.19.9)
2. *Sopakramaṃ nirupakramaṃ ca karma tatsaṃyamādaparāntajñānam.* (सोपक्रमं निरुपक्रमं च कर्म तत्संयमादपरान्तज्ञानम्॥) (Y.S. III.21)
3. *"Ito tiṇṇaṃ māsānaṃ accayena tathāgato parinibbāyissati."* ("इतो तिण्णं मासानं अच्चयेन तथागतो परिनिब्बायिस्सति।") (Dīgha. Mahāvaggo दीघ० । महावग्गो । 3.17.56)
4. *Kāyarūpasaṃyamāttadgrāhyaśaktistambhe cakṣuḥprakāśāsamprayoge' ntardhānam.* (कायरूपसंयमात्तद्ग्राह्यशक्तिस्तम्भे चक्षुःप्रकाशासंप्रयोगेऽन्तर्धानम्॥) (Y.S. III. 20)
5. *Dhammiyā kathāya sandassetvā . . . antaradhāyāmi, antarahitaṃ ca maṃ na jānanti – 'ko nu kho ayaṃ antarahito devo vā manusso vā', ti?* (धम्मिया कथाय सन्दस्सेत्वा....अन्तरधायामि। अन्तरहितं च मं न जानन्ति 'को नु खो अयं अन्तरहितो देवो वा मनुस्सो वा' ति?) (Dīgha. Mahāvaggo दीघ० ।

• Celestial temptations –

Patanjali warns against celestial temptations, that is, temptations proceeding from divine beings.[1]

Māra (मार), the Tempter, tried to seduce the Buddha on numerous occasions but always failed in his objective. His daughters *Taṇhā* (तण्हा), *Arati* (अरति) and *Ragā* (रगा) also tried to seduce him after his Enlightenment but in vain.[2]

Pali texts mention many occasions on which *Māra* would assume various forms to tempt nuns (*bhikkhunī-s*) (भिक्खुनी), often in lonely spots.[3]

• Importance of 'Practice' (*abhyāsa*) (अभ्यास) for developing 'Stationary Samādhi'–

After describing the five kinds of mental processes, the Yoga-Sutras lay down that their restraint is produced by means of Practice (*abhyāsa*) (अभ्यास) and Detachment (*vairāgya*) (वैराग्य).[4] Out of these, *abhyāsa* (अभ्यास) means effort for stability (*sthiti*) (स्थिति) (of the mind)[5] which becomes firm when it is cultivated for a long time, uninterruptedly and with earnest attention.[6]

The use of the word *sthiti* (स्थिति) (Pali *ṭhiti*) (ठिति) as above seems to allude to the development of *ṭhitibhāgiyo samādhi*

महावग्गो । 3.12.42)

1. *Sthānyupanimantraṇe saṅgasmayākaraṇaṃ punariṣṭaprasaṅgāt.* (स्थान्युपनिमन्त्रणे सङ्गस्मयाकरणं पुनरिष्टप्रसङ्गात् ॥) (Y.S. III. 51)
2. *Saṃyutta, Māradhītusuttaṃ.* (संयुत्त०, मारधीतुसुत्तं – 4.25.34.)
3. *Āḷavikā* (आळविका), *Somā* (सोमा), *Gotamī* (गोतमी), *Vijayā* (विजया), *Uppalavaṇṇā* (उप्पलवण्णा), to quote a few. *(Saṃyutta. Bhikkhunī-saṃyuttaṃ* -संयुत्त० । भिक्खुनीसंयुत्तं ।)
4. *Abhyāsavairāgyābhyāṃ tannirodhaḥ.* (अभ्यासवैराग्याभ्यां तन्निरोधः ॥) (Y.S. I.12)
5. *Tatra sthitau yatno' bhyāsaḥ.* (तत्र स्थितौ यत्नोऽभ्यासः ॥) (Y.S. I.13)
6. *Sa tu dīrghakālanairantaryasatkārāsevito dṛḍhabhūmiḥ.* (स तु दीर्घकालनैरन्तर्यसत्काराऽऽसेवितो दृढभूमिः ॥) (Y.S. I.14)

(ठितिभागियो समाधि) (that is, stationary *samādhi*) met with in the Buddha's expositions, the other three types being *hānabhāgiyo* (हानभागियो) (declining *samādhi*), *visesabhāgiyo* (विसेसभागियो) (distinctive *samādhi*, leading to the attainment of various super-normal powers) and *nibbedhabhāgiyo* (निब्बेधभागियो) (penetrating *samādhi*).[1]

For the attainment of stationary *samādhi*, one has to practise continuously and uninterruptedly which, depending upon the earnestness of the practitioner, results in the cultivation of *khaṇika samādhi* (खणिक समाधि) (concentration sustained from moment to moment), *upacāra samādhi* (उपचार समाधि) (neighbourhood concentration, of a level approaching a state of absorption) or *appanā samādhi* (अप्पना समाधि) (attainment concentration, a state of mental absorption, i.e., *jhāna* (झान)), in that order.

In Pali texts the general word used for denoting a person established in *samādhi* (समाधि) is *patiṭṭhito* (पतिट्ठितो) (Skt. *pratiṣṭhitaḥ*) (प्रतिष्ठितः).[2]

• Importance of 'Detachment' (*vairāgya*) (वैराग्य) in curbing mental processes –

According to Yoga-Sutras, 'Detachment' (*vairāgya*) (वैराग्य) is one of the factors which helps in curbing mental processes.[3]

For the Buddha, of all the laws 'Detachment' (*virāga*) (विराग) stood at the top.[4]

---

1. *Paṭisambhidā* (पटिसम्भिदा०) 1.1.3.106
2. *Catūsu satipaṭṭhānesu supatiṭṭhitacitto* (चतूसु सतिपट्ठानेसु सुपतिट्ठितचित्तो०) (Dīgha. Mahāvaggo दीघ० । महावग्गो । 3.4.16)
3. Y.S. I. 12
4. *Yāvatā, bhikkhave, dhammā saṅkhatā vā asaṅkhatā vā, virāgo tesaṃ aggamakkhāyati.* (यावता, भिक्खवे, धम्मा सङ्खता वा असङ्खता वा, विरागो तेसं अग्गमक्खायति ।) (Itivuttaka. इतिवुत्तक - 3.41.43)

• Ecstatic States: *samādhi-s* (समाधि) and *jhāna-s* (झान) –

Patanjali refers to two types of concentration (*samādhi-s*) (समाधि), the first one called *samprajñāta* (सम्प्रज्ञात) (i.e., with intuitive knowledge) and the second one simply called *anya* (अन्य) (i.e., another).

The first one has for its concomitants *vitarka, vicāra, ānanda* (वितर्क, विचार, आनन्द) and *asmitā* (अस्मिता) (i.e., initial application of mind to the object, sustained attention to the object, joy or bliss and sense-of-personality).[1] For the other one it has been mentioned that it requires effort for experiencing cessation (of cognition) and in this only a subliminal impression forms the residue.[2]

Before becoming a fully enlightened person, the Buddha had learnt and practised the eight Absorptions (*jhāna-s*) (झान)[3] prevalent in those days. The first four of them are called *rūpajjhāna-s* (रूपज्झान), achieved through the attainment of full concentration (*appanā samādhi*) (अप्पना समाधि). In these there is a complete, though temporary, suspension of the fivefold sense-activity and of the five Hindrances (*nīvaraṇa-s*) (नीवरण).[4] The state of consciousness, however, is one of alertness and lucidity.

The first Absorption is accompanied by *vitakka, vicāra, pīti, sukha* (वितक्क, विचार, पीति, सुख) and *cittekaggatā* (चित्तेकग्गता) (i.e., initial application of mind to the object, sustained

---

1. *Vitarkavicārānandāsmitārūpānugamāt samprajñātaḥ.* (वितर्कविचारानन्दास्मितारूपानुगमात्सम्प्रज्ञातः ॥) (Y.S. I.17)
2. *Virāmapratyayābhyāsapūrvaḥ saṃskāraśeṣo' nyaḥ.* (विरामप्रत्ययाभ्यासपूर्वः संस्कारशेषोऽन्यः ॥) (Y.S. I.18)
3. *Skt. dhyāna* (ध्यान)
4. *Kāmacchanda, byāpāda, thinamiddha, uddhaccakukkucca, vicikicchā.* (कामच्छन्द, ब्यापाद, थिनमिद्ध, उद्धच्चकुक्कुच्च, विचिकिच्छा) (i.e., Sensuous Desire, Ill-will, Sloth and Torpor, Restlessness and Scruples, Sceptical Doubt).

attention to the object, joy, bliss and concentration of mind).[1] The second Absorption is accompanied by *pīti, sukha* (पीति, सुख) and *ekaggatā* (एकग्गता) (i.e., joy, bliss and concentration of mind), the remaining two having subsided. The third Absorption is accompanied by *sukha* (सुख) and *cittekaggatā* (चित्तेकग्गता) (i.e., bliss and concentration of mind), *pīti* (पीति) (i.e., joy) having subsided. The fourth Absorption is accompanied by only *cittekaggatā* (चित्तेकग्गता) (i.e., concentration of mind), *sukha* (सुख) (i.e., bliss) having subsided.

The next four Absorptions are known as *arūpajjhāna-s* (अरूपज्झान) which enable one to enter the realms of infinity of space *(ākāsānañcāyatanasamāpatti)* (आकासानञ्चायतनसमापत्ति), infinity of consciousness *(viññāṇañcāyatanasamāpatti)* (विञ्ञाणञ्चायतनसमापत्ति), nothingness *(ākiñcaññāyatanasamāpatti)* (आकिञ्चञ्ञायतनसमापत्ति) and neither perception nor yet non-perception *(nevasaññānāsaññāyatanasamāpatti)* (नेवसञ्ञानासञ्ञायतनसमापत्ति).

The difference in the two sets of Absorptions is that in the first four one remains in the field of mind and matter while in the last four only the mind functions. Even having experienced all these eight Absorptions, the Buddha discovered that they could not eliminate from his psyche the deep-rooted mental defilements (*anusaya kilesa-s*) (अनुसय किलेस). He, therefore, decided to practise on his own and discovered the path which led to 'the cessation of perception and sensations' called *saññāvedayitanirodha* (सञ्ञावेदयितनिरोध) or *nirodhasamāpatti* (निरोधसमापत्ति), or simply *nirodha* (निरोध). This was a stage in which even mind (*citta*) (चित्त) ceased to function and one experienced the state of liberation (*nibbāna*) (निब्बान). The Buddha became a *buddha* (बुद्ध) only after he had made this

1. *Paṭhamaṃ jhānaṃ paṭilābhatthāya vitakko ca vicāro ca pīti ca sukhaṃ ca cittekaggatā ca* . . . (पठमं झानं पटिलाभत्थाय वितक्को च विचारो च पीति च सुखं च चित्तेकग्गता च.......।) (Paṭisambhidā. पटिसम्भिदा० – 1.5.0.2.2.9)

discovery. Before this, he was only a *bodhisatta* (बोधिसत्त), that is, one striving to become a Buddha.

The discovery made by the Buddha was that it was not essential to practise the eight Absorptions for experiencing the state of liberation. For this, recourse could be had only to the first four with the modification that one might introduce an element of detachment (*viveka*) (विवेक) from the very first Absorption which would induce deep concentration (*samādhi*) (समाधि) in the second and pave the way for mindfulness and constant thorough realization of mind-matter phenomena (*sati-sampajañña*) (सति-सम्पजञ्ञ) in the third. In the culmination of this Absorption, the twin faculties of *sati-sampajañña* (सति-सम्पजञ्ञ) would become so strong that one would not forsake them even for a moment.[1] Having reached this stage when one enters the fourth Absorption there is simultaneous experience of fruit of liberation (*phala-samāpatti*) (फलसमापत्ति) with the experience of perfect concentration (*jhāna-samāpatti*) (झानसमापत्ति). This is a special feature of the Buddha's technique of meditation and has been extolled highly in one of his most important *sutta-s*.[2]

For Patanjali *samprajñāta samādhi* (सम्प्रज्ञात समाधि) (concentration with intuitive knowledge) is one which is accompanied by *vitarka* (वितर्क), *vicāra* (विचार), *ānanda* (आनन्द) and *asmitā* (अस्मिता) (i.e., initial application of mind to the object, sustained attention to the object, joy or bliss and sense-of-personality) which is, more or less, compatible with

1. *Yato ca bhikkhu ātāpi, sampajaññaṃ na riñcati.* (यतो च भिक्खु आतापि, सम्पजञ्ञं न रिञ्चति।) (Saṃyutta. संयुत्त॰ 36.12.12)
2. *Yaṃ buddhaseṭṭho parivaṇṇayī suciṃ, samādhimānantarikaññamāhu. Samādhinā tena samo na vijjati, idampi dhamme ratanaṃ paṇītaṃ.* (यं बुद्धसेट्ठो परिवण्णयी सुचिं, समाधिमानन्तरिकञ्ञमाहु। समाधिना तेन समो न विज्जति, इदम्पि धम्मे रतनं पणीतं॥) (Khuddaka. (खुद्दक) – 6.5)

the Buddha's teaching. The other *samādhi anyaḥ* (अन्य:),[1] which aims at the cessation (*virāma*) (विराम) or *nirodha* (निरोध) of cognitions and has a residue of subliminal impression (*saṃskāra*) (संस्कार) is also compatible as this seems to relate to the stage of a *sotāpanna* (सोतापन्न) (Stream-enterer) who, too, experiences cessation of perception and sensations (*saññāvedayita-nirodha*) (सञ्ञावेदयितनिरोध) and has just a few subliminal impressions (*saṅkhāra-s*) (सङ्खार) of higher planes of consciousness to get rid of before attaining the state of Arahanthood.

It will, thus, be seen that, in essence, Patanjali's teaching is quite compatible with the Buddha's but, in later times, this aspect was lost sight of because of the fanciful interpretations of his commentators.

• Selection of a befitting subject for concentration of mind –

After giving a few instances of what might serve as subjects fit for concentration of the mind, the Yoga-Sutras also enjoin that one may select a subject of one's own choice.[2]

According to the Buddha's teaching also, one may apprehend from amongst the forty meditation subjects[3] prescribed for mundane concentration any one that suits one's temperament. The six kinds of temperaments recognised were

---

1. Improperly called *asaṃprajñāta* 'असम्प्रज्ञात' by Patanjali's commentators: this could have been called *saṃprajñānātīta* 'सम्प्रज्ञानातीत' which would have been a more apt nomenclature, consistent with its actual description.
2. *Yathābhimatadhyānād vā.* (यथाभिमतध्यानाद् वा ॥) (Y.S. I.39)
3. *Tatrimāni cattālīsa kammaṭṭhānāni: dasa kasiṇā, dasa asubhā, dasa anussastiyo, cattāro brahmavihārā, cattāro āruppā, ekā saññā, ekaṃ vavatthānaṃ ti.* (तत्रिमानि चत्तालीस कम्मट्ठानानि: दस कसिणा, दस असुभा, दस अनुस्सतियो, चत्तारो ब्रह्मविहारा, चत्तारो आरुप्पा, एका सञ्ञा, एकं ववत्थानं ति) (Visuddhi. विसुद्धि० - III. 104)

greedy, hating, deluded, faithful, intelligent and speculative.[1]

• The distractions of the mind: *Cittavikṣepāḥ* (चित्तविक्षेपाः) –

According to the Yoga-Sutras, the distractions of the mind are: ailment, langour, doubt, carelessness, sloth, sensuality, erratic perception, missing the ground and instability. These are the obstacles.[2]

Barring ailment (*vyādhi*) (व्याधि), which had been dealt with separately in detail by the Buddha, the other distractions of the mind *(cittavikṣepāḥ)* (चित्तविक्षेपा:) were also spelt out by him.

Byādhi (ब्याधि) is to be realised as suffering *(dukkha)* (दुक्ख) and its opposite *A-byādhi* as pleasure (*sukha*) (सुख). *Byādhi* is to be realised as fear (*bhaya*) (भय) and *A-byādhi* as security (*khema*) (खेम). *Byādhi* is to be realised as something composed (*saṅkhāra*) (सङ्खार) and *A-byādhi* as total extinction (*nibbāna*) (निब्बान).[3]

The remaining distractions of the mind listed by Patanjali are covered in the Buddha's lore in the following manner:

Styāna (स्त्यान) (langour) as *thina* (थिन); *saṃśaya* (संशय) (doubt) as *vicikicchā* (विचिकिच्छा); *pramāda* (प्रमाद)

1. *Rāgacariyā, dosacariyā, mohacariyā, saddhācariyā, buddhicariyā, vitakkacariyā.* (रागचरिया, दोसचरिया, मोहचरिया, सद्धाचरिया, बुद्धिचरिया, वितक्कचरिया) । (Visuddhi. विसुद्धि० – III. 74)
2. *Vyādhistyānasaṃśayapramādālasyāviratibhrāntidarśanā-labdhabhūmikatvānavasthitatvāni cittavikṣepāste'ntarāyāḥ.* (व्याधिस्त्यानसंशयप्रमादालस्याविरतिभ्रान्तिदर्शनालब्धभूमिकत्वानवस्थितत्वानि चित्तविक्षेपास्तेऽन्तरायाः ॥) (Y.S. I.30)
3. *Byādhi dukkhaṃ, abyādhi sukhaṃ ti abhiññeyyaṃ. Byādhi bhayaṃ, abyādhi khemaṃ ti abhiññeyyaṃ. Byādhi saṅkhārā, abyādhi nibbānaṃ ti abhiññeyyaṃ.* (ब्याधि दुक्खं, अब्याधि सुखं ति अभिञ्ञेय्यं। ब्याधि भयं, अब्याधि खेमं ति अभिञ्ञेय्यं। ब्याधि सङ्खारा, अब्याधि निब्बानं ति अभिञ्ञेय्यं।) (Paṭisambhidā. पटिसम्भिदा० 1.1.1.25, 26, 28).

(carelessness) as *kosajja* (कोसज्ज); *ālasya* (आलस्य) (sloth) as *middha* (मिद्ध); *avirati* (अविरति) (sensuality) as *rāga* (राग); *bhrāntidarśana* (भ्रान्तिदर्शन) (erratic perception) as *avijjā* (अविज्जा); *alabdhabhūmikatva* (अलब्धभूमिकत्व) (missing the ground) as *atītānudhāvana* and *anāgatapaṭikaṅkhana citta* (अतीतानुधावन, अनागतपटिकङ्खन चित्त); and *anavasthitatva* (अनवस्थितत्व) (instability) as *kukkucca* (कुक्कुच्च).[1]

• Concomitants of the dispersions of the mind –

In the Yoga-Sutras it has been mentioned that suffering (*duḥkha*) (दु:ख), mental un-ease (*daurmanasya*) (दौर्मनस्य), agitation of the body (*aṅgamejayatva*) (अङ्गमेजयत्व), inspiration (*śvāsa*) (श्वास) and expiration (*praśvāsa*) (प्रश्वास) are the concomitants of the dispersions of the mind (*vikṣepasahabhuvaḥ*) (विक्षेपसहभुव:).[2] And to ward these off, effort for stability on a single entity must be practised.[3]

While practising Vipassanā - the technique of meditation taught by the Buddha—one discovers at the experiential level that with every disturbance in the mind there follow, as a corrollary, pain in the form of some unpleasant sensation,

---

1. *Atītānudhāvanaṃ cittaṃ vikkhepānupatitaṃ - samādhisssa paripantho. Anāgatapaṭikaṅkhanaṃ cittaṃ vikampitaṃ - samādhissa paripantho. Līnaṃ cittaṃ kosajjānupatitaṃ - samādhissa paripantho. Abhinataṃ cittaṃ rāgānupatitaṃ - samādhissa paripantho.* (अतीतानुधावनं चित्तं विक्खेपानुपतितं - समाधिस्स परिपन्थो। अनागत-पटिकङ्खनं चित्तं विकम्पितं - समाधिस्स परिपन्थो। लीनं चित्तं कोसज्जानुपतितं - समाधिस्स परिपन्थो। अभिनतं चित्तं रागानुपतितं - समाधिस्स परिपन्थो।) (Paṭisambhidā पटिसम्भिदा॰ 1.3.2.8) And, *thinamiddhaṃ nīvaraṇaṃ, . . . kukkuccaṃ nīvaraṇaṃ, vicikicchā nīvaraṇaṃ, avijjā nīvaraṇaṃ.* (थिनमिद्धं नीवरणं, ... कुक्कुच्चं नीवरणं, विचिकिच्छा नीवरणं, अविज्जा नीवरणं.....।) (Paṭisambhidā. पटिसम्भिदा॰ 1.3.1.4)
2. *Duḥkhadaurmanasyāṅgamejayatva-śvāsapraśvāsā vikṣepasahabhuvaḥ.* (दु:खदौर्मनस्याङ्गमेजयत्वश्वासप्रश्वासा विक्षेपसहभुव: ॥) (Y.S. I.31)
3. *Tatpratiṣedhārthamekatatvābhyāsaḥ.* (तत्प्रतिषेधार्थमेकतत्त्वाभ्यास: ॥) (Y.S. I.32)

mental un-ease, agitation of body and change in the normal flow of respiration. So far as the agitation of the body and mental un-ease are concerned, the Buddha ordained: "Oh meditators, when concentration on mindfulness is practised several times the swaying motion of the body or the mind does not take place."[1]

• The doctrine of not-self (*Anātmabhāva*) (अनात्मभाव) –

Patanjali affirms that the notion of self (*ātmabhāva*) (आत्मभाव) ceases for him who sees in a special way (*viśeṣadarśinaḥ*) (विशेषदर्शिन:).[2]

This seems to be an unmistakable reference to *Vipassanā* (विपस्सना), the technique of insight-meditation taught by the Buddha. *Vipassanā* (विपस्सना) (also known as *vidarśanā* (विदर्शना) means 'to see things in a special way (that is, the correct way—not as they appear to be, but as they really are as ultimate reality)'. Thus, the prefix *vi* (वि) in *Vipassanā* or *vidarśanā* (विदर्शना) stands for *viśeṣa* (विशेष) (special).[3] A *Viśeṣadarśī* (विशेषदर्शी) is, accordingly, a Vipassanā meditator who has learnt how to see things in a special way.

As one practises the technique of Vipassanā meditation, one begins to feel the arising and passing away of the mind-matter phenomena at the experiential level. With further

---

1. *"Ānāpānassatisamādhissa, bhikkhave, bhāvitattā bahulīkatattā neva kāyassa iñjitattaṃ vā hoti phanditattaṃ vā, na cittassa iñjitattaṃ vā hoti phanditattaṃ vā."* ("आनापानस्सतिसमाधिस्स, भिक्खवे, भावितत्ता बहुलीकतत्ता नेव कायस्स इञ्जितत्तं वा होति फन्दितत्तं वा, न चित्तस्स इञ्जितत्तं वा होति फन्दितत्तं वा।") (Saṃyutta. संयुत्त० – 54.7.7)
2. *Viśeṣadarśinaḥ ātmabhāvabhāvanāvinivṛttiḥ.* (विशेषदर्शिन: आत्मभावभावनाविनिवृत्तिः ॥) (Y.S. IV.25)
3. *Paññattiṃ ṭhapetvā visesena passatī ti vipassanā.* (पञ्ञत्तिं ठपेत्वा विसेसेन पस्सतीति विपस्सना।) (Nettipakaraṇa, Aṭṭhakathā (नेत्तिपकरण अट्ठकथा), (p. 133, Burmese edition) that is, seeing (experience of the reality) in a special way, by disintegrating the apparent truth (working towards the ultimate truth) is *Vipassanā.*

growth in this technique one begins to have such an experience at all times and in all situations. At this stage the meditator begins to realise that his physical structure is not "I", not "mine" and is devoid of any self or substance. Similarly, his mental structure is not "I", not "mine" and is devoid of any self or substance.[1] Thus, the deep-rooted notion of there being a self within the framework of the body (or, for that matter, within the phenomenal world) begins to melt away with the practice of Vipassanā.

While the other teachings of the Buddha may, more or less, be found ingrained in many philosophical systems and religions of India, *anattā* (अनत्ता) has been clearly and un-reservedly taught by him alone.[2] It is for this reason that he is known as *anattā-vādī* (अनत्ता-वादी) or the Teacher of Impersonality. Hence Patanjali's reference to the notion of self (*ātmabhāva*) (आत्मभाव) ceasing for one who sees in a special way (*viśeṣadarśinaḥ*) (विशेषदर्शिन:) speaks volumes for his appreciation of Vipassanā as a result-oriented technique of meditation.

- **'Purity of mindfulness' (*smṛtipariśuddhi*) (स्मृतिपरिशुद्धि) and the induction of balanced states –**

This topic is broached by Patanjali in two of his aphorisms[3] which are generally translated as:

---

1. *'Netaṃ mama, nesohamasmi, na meso attā' ti* ('नेतं मम, नेसोहमस्मि, न मेसो अत्ता' ति) । (Saṃyutta. संयुत्त० – 22.59.62)
2. '. . . *whether Perfect Ones arise or do not arise the characteristics of impermanence and pain are made known, but unless there is the arising of a Buddha the characteristic of not-self is not made known.*' (*Vibhaṅga Aṭṭhakathā* विभङ्ग अट्ठकथा 49-50)
3. *Smṛtipariśuddhau svarūpaśūnyevārthamātranirbhāsā nirvitarkā. Etayaiva savicārā nirvicārā ca sūkṣmaviṣayā vyākhyātā.* (स्मृतिपरिशुद्धौ स्वरूपशून्येवार्थमात्रनिर्भासा निर्वितर्का॥ एतयैव सविचारा निर्विचारा च सूक्ष्मविषया व्याख्याता॥) (Y.S. I.43, 44)

"When mindfulness is purified, the shining of the object alone (in the mind), which appears as if it is not there, is the (balanced state) without application of mind to the object (*nirvitarkā*) (निर्वितर्का). By this, the (balanced states) with sustained attention to the object (*savicārā*) (सविचारा) as also without sustained attention to the object (*nirvicārā*) (निर्विचारा) having subtle objects (as their support) stand explained."

A close examination of these aphorisms would show that these echo the Buddha's teaching. According to the Buddha, all *vitakka-s* (वितक्क) and *vicāra-s* (विचार) are due to one's Ego (i.e., the false notion of "I', "Me", "Mine", etc.). Patanjali refers to this as *swa-rūpa* (स्व-रूप), i.e., one's entity, which in other words means *ātma-bhāva* (आत्म-भाव)—*atta-bhāva* (अत्त-भाव) in Buddha's terminology. As soon as this melts away, one attains the balanced states which are free from *vitakka-s* (वितक्क) and *vicāra-s* (विचार). On reaching these states, when one says "I", "Me", "Mine", one realizes that this is for the sake of (worldly) dealings (*arthamātranirbhāsā*) (अर्थमात्रनिर्भासा) that these words are used, otherwise they are meaningless.[1]

The term *upekkhā-sati-pārisuddhiṃ* (उपेक्खा-सति-पारिसुद्धिं) occurs in the context of the fourth Absorption in the Buddha's famous discourse known as *Mahāsatipaṭṭhāna-Sutta* (महासतिपट्ठान-सुत्त).[2] This means 'with purity of equanimity and mindfulness.' Both the teachers—Patanjali and the Buddha—recognise the importance of 'purity of mindfulness' in attaining the balanced states of mind free from initial

1. This applies squarely to an arahant who uses such expressions only for the sake of worldly dealings.
Cf. Yo hoti bhikkhu arahaṃ katāvī . . . ahaṃ vadāmītipi so vadeyya. mamaṃ vadantītipi so vadeyya, loke samaññaṃ kusalo viditvā, vohāramattena so vohareyya. (यो होति भिक्खु अरहं कतावी ..... अहं वदामीतिपि सो वदेय्य, ममं वदन्तीतिपि सो वदेय्य, लोके समञ्ञं कुसलो विदित्वा, वोहारमत्तेन सो वोहरेय्य।) (Saṃyutta. संयुत्त॰ 1.25.31)
2. "*. . . adukkhamasukhaṃ upekkhāsatipārisuddhiṃ catutthaṃ jhānaṃ upasampajja viharati.*" (".... अदुक्खमसुखं उपेक्खासतिपारिसुद्धिं चतुत्थं झानं उपसम्पज्ज विहरति") (Dīgha, Mahāvaggo. दीघ॰ । महावग्गो । 9.5.31)

application of mind to the object (*vitarka-s*) (वितर्क) and sustained attention to the object (*vicāra-s*) (विचार), in other words, free from Ego-ism. The Buddha declared that one could come out of 'ego-ism' completely through the constant practice of the "Four-fold Satipaṭṭhāna" taught by him.

The "Four-fold Satipaṭṭhāna" has *sampajañña* (सम्पजञ्ञ) (constant thorough realisation of impermanence of mind-matter phenomena) as its essential ingredient. *Sampajañña* (सम्पजञ्ञ) is for experiencing impermanence (*aniccatā*) (अनिच्चता). This experience of impermanence has to be developed for dispelling belief in one's personality. When this belief is dispelled, one attains the state of *nibbāna* in this very life.[1]

• Misconception relating to Perceiver, Perceptivity and Perception –

In the Yoga-Sutras an attempt has been made to resolve the misconception relating to Perceiver (*draṣṭā*) (द्रष्टा), Perceptivity (*darśana*) (दर्शन) and Perception (*dṛśya*) (दृश्य). Stating that for the discriminant there is nothing but misery in this world,[2] Patanjali counsels that one may try to avoid the misery that has not yet befallen.[3] He explains that the cause of such misery is the conjunction (*saṃyoga*) (संयोग) of the Perceiver (*draṣṭā*) (द्रष्टा) with Perceptivity (*darśana*) (दर्शन).[4] The Perceiver ultimately manifests itself merely as Pure

---

1. *Aniccasaññā bhāvetabbā asmimānasamugghātāya. Aniccasaññino hi, Meghiya, anattasaññā saṇṭhāti, anattasaññī asmimānasamugghātaṃ pāpuṇāti diṭṭheva dhamme nibbānaṃ.* (अनिच्चसञ्ञा भावेतब्बा अस्मिमानसमुग्घाताय। अनिच्चसञ्ञिनो हि, मेघिय, अनत्तसञ्ञा सण्ठाति, अनत्तसञ्ञी अस्मिमानसमुग्घातं पापुणाति दिट्ठेव धम्मे निब्बानं।) (Udāna. उदान 4.1.4)
2. *Duḥkhameva sarvaṃ vivekinaḥ* (दुःखमेव सर्वं विवेकिनः॥) (Y.S. II. 15)
3. *Heyaṃ duḥkhamanāgatam.* (हेयं दुःखमनागतम्॥) (Y.S. II.16)
4. *Draṣṭṛdṛśyayoḥ saṃyogo heyahetuḥ.* (द्रष्टृदृश्ययोः संयोगो हेयहेतुः॥) (Y.S. II.17)

Consciousness (*dṛśi*) (दृशि) but, though pure (*śuddho'pi*) (शुद्धोऽपि), its cause (*pratyaya*) (प्रत्यय), nevertheless, still remains to be introspected minutely (*anupaśyaḥ*) (अनुपश्यः).[1] The semblance of Perception (*dṛśya*) (दृश्य) is only for this purpose.[2] The cause of conjunction (which has been shown above to be the cause of misery) is Ignorance (*avidyā*) (अविद्या).[3] When Ignorance is dissipated, the Conjunction also gets dissipated; this is the falling apart (*hānaṃ*) (हानं). That constitutes the isolation of Pure Consciousness (*tad dṛśeḥ kaivalyam* (तद् दृशेः कैवल्यम्).[4] The means of this falling apart is the un-wavering Discriminating Knowledge (*vivekakhyātiḥ*) (विवेकख्यातिः).[5]

All these statements made by Patanjali conform to the Buddha's teaching which has for its basis the technique of Vipassanā meditation. 'Vipassanā' (विपस्सना) is a technique of self-realisation, investigating the reality of what one calls oneself. One gets direct experience of this reality by focussing one's attention from superficial, apparent, gross reality to subtler realities and, eventually, the subtlest reality of mind and matter. Having experienced all these, one goes further to experience the Ultimate Reality which is beyond mind and matter.

In this process of self-realisation one discovers that within the physical and mental structure there is no "I", no "mine". The entire phenomenon is nothing but 'vibrations' which do not last more than a moment. Then the misconception that there is a Perceiver (*draṣṭā*) (द्रष्टा) or Perception (*dṛśya*) (दृश्य) in the mind-matter phenomena is dispelled. At an intermediate

---

1. *Draṣṭā dṛśimātraḥ śuddho'pi pratyayānupaśyaḥ.* (द्रष्टा दृशिमात्रः शुद्धोऽपि प्रत्ययानुपश्यः ॥) (Y.S. II. 20)
2. *Tadartha eva dṛśyasyātmā.* (तदर्थ एव दृश्यस्यात्मा ॥) (Y.S. II. 21)
3. *Tasya heturavidyā.* (तस्य हेतुरविद्या) (Y.S. II. 24)
4. *Tadabhāvātsaṃyogābhāvo hānaṃ tad dṛśeḥ kaivalyam.* (तदभावात्संयोगाभावो हानं तद् दृशेः कैवल्यम्) (Y.S. II.25)
5. *Vivekakhyātiraviplavā hānopāyaḥ.* (विवेकख्यातिरविप्लवा हानोपायः ॥) (Y.S. II.26)

stage of self-realisation, one becomes aware of Pure Consciousness alone as a stark reality. When Patanjali speaks of '*draṣṭā dṛśimātraḥ*' (द्रष्टा दृशिमात्रः) he seems to be referring to this stage of there being no entity to be called a Perceiver (*draṣṭā*) (द्रष्टा) and that Pure Consciousness alone holds the field.

In the technique of Vipassanā meditation, this is a very important stage because one's mindfulness remains confined to 'pure consciousness' (*viññāṇa*) (विञ्ञाण) (Skt. *vijñāna*) (विज्ञान). But still curiosity arises as to what might be the cause (*pratyaya*) (प्रत्यय) of even this 'pure consciousness' (*viññāṇa*) (विञ्ञाण). To arrive at the truth, one has to resort to minute introspection (*anupaśyanā*) (अनुपश्यना) even of this phenomenon. When this is done, one begins to experience six different types of consciousness, each according to its relationship with a particular sense-door. Thus, Pure Consciousness (*viññāṇa*) (विञ्ञाण) is cognised as consciousness distinctly related either to eye, or ear, or nose, or tongue, or skin, or mind. One learns from experience that these different types come into existence as soon as there is contact (*phassa*) (फस्स) or conjunction (*saṃyoga*) (संयोग) of a sense-door with its respective object. Further introspection of this phenomenon reveals that the sense-doors as well as their objects are simply in the nature of subtle vibrations which just arise and pass away. Thus, the entire physical structure as well as the mental structure is experienced as nothing but subtle vibrations. With such an experience, the notion of there being a Self (*i.e.*, a permanently abiding principle) within is completely dispelled.

Till such time as one undergoes such an experience, one remains ignorant of the reality pertaining to the mind-matter phenomena and keeps on generating misery for oneself by building *saṅkhāra-s* (सङ्खार) (Skt. *saṃskāra-s*) (संस्कार) by reacting in different situations of life. Patanjali has rightly pointed out, in line with the Buddha's exposition, that the isolation of Pure Consciousness (*dṛśeḥ kaivalyaṃ*) (दृशेः कैवल्यं)

comes about when the conjunction of the Perceiver and Perception (*draṣṭṛdṛśyayoḥ saṃyogaḥ*) (द्रष्टृदृश्ययोः संयोगः) — which is the cause of misery—falls apart through minute introspection (*anupaśyanā*) (अनुपश्यना). The process which enables one to achieve this objective has been referred to by Patanjali as *vivekakhyāti* (विवेकख्याति) (that is, perception based upon discrimination). This seems to be another name for *vipassanā* (विपस्सना), which is also definable as *vivekena passatī ti* (विवेकेन पस्सती ति) (*i.e.*, a technique enabling one to perceive things with discrimination).

When one becomes adept in *vivekakhyāti* (विवेकख्याति) (or, *vipassanā* विपस्सना), one starts realising at the experiential level how consciousness (*viññāṇa*) (विञ्ञाण) arises and passes away at every perception through the various senses. Thus, 'seeing' remains confined to 'seeing', 'hearing' to 'hearing', 'smelling' to 'smelling', 'tasting' to 'tasting', 'touching' to 'touching' and 'cognition' to 'cognition'[1]. Further introspection dissolves even this awareness into subtle vibrations at every sense-door and everywhere else.

The functions of *vivekakhyāti* (विवेकख्याति) and *vipassanā* (विपस्सना) are one and the same, viz., to enable one to realise the ultimate truth by disintegrating the apparent truth. The Buddha's methodology is known as *vibhajjavāda* (विभज्जवाद), that is to say, a methodology by means of which one keeps on analysing phenomena till the ultimate truth is revealed.[2]

1. On this the Buddha's words are—*"Diṭṭhe diṭṭhamattaṃ bhavissati, sute sutamattaṃ bhavissati, mute mutamattaṃ bhavissati, viññāte viññātamattaṃ bhavissati"* ("दिट्ठे दिट्ठमत्तं भविस्सति, सुते सुतमत्तं भविस्सति, मुते मुतमत्तं भविस्सति, विञ्ञाते विञ्ञातमत्तं भविस्सति।") (Udāna. उदान – 1.10.21)
2. *"Vibhajjavādo kho ahamettha, māṇava . . .* "(विभज्जवादो खो अहमेत्थ, माणव...) Majjhima. Majjhima – paṇṇāsakaṃ (मज्झिम.। मज्झिम-पण्णासकं) 49.1.2

• The concept of 'Dharma-megha'—

In the Yoga-Sutras a reference has been made to a *samādhi* called '*dharmamegha*' (धर्ममेघ). It is attained by one who, strenuous even while working in the higher states of meditation in the realm of mind and matter (*i.e.*, the sensory field), keeps on making use of discriminative knowledge in every way.[1] From this follows the cessation of hindrances and Karma.[2] Then, because of the boundlessness of knowledge which stands freed from all covering defilements, what remains yet to be known amounts to very little.[3]

In the Buddha's lore, there is no *samādhi* (समाधि) called *dhammamegha* (धम्ममेघ) (Skt. *dharmamegha*) (धर्ममेघ), although the use of this word is met with in connection with the dissolution of defiling impulses (*āsava-s*) (आसव):

"While the *dhammamegha* keeps raining, may all be free from their defiling impulses (*anāsavā*) (अनासवा). May such of the persons present here who (because of their rich *pāramitā-s* of the past) are in the final phase of their mundane existence become at least Stream-enterers (*sotāpanna*) (सोतापन्न)![4]

A person becomes a Stream-enterer only after the disappearance of the three fetters of personality-belief, sceptical doubt and attachment to rules and rituals. Because of his entry into the stream leading to *nibbāna* (निब्बान) (Final Emancipation), he is no more subject to re-birth in the lower worlds, is firmly established in Dhamma and is destined to

---

1. *Prasaṅkhyāne' pyakusīdasya sarvathā vivekakhyāterdharmameghaḥ samādhiḥ.* (प्रसङ्ख्यानेऽप्यकुसीदस्य सर्वथा विवेकख्यातेर्धर्ममेघः समाधिः ॥) (Y.S. IV. 29)
2. *Tataḥ kleśakarmanivṛttiḥ.* (ततः क्लेशकर्मनिवृत्तिः ॥) (Y.S. IV.30)
3. *Tadā sarvāvaraṇamalāpetasya jñānasyānantyājjñeyamalpam.* (तदा सर्वावरणमलापेतस्य ज्ञानस्यानन्त्याज्ज्ञेयमल्पम् ॥) (Y.S. IV.31)
4. *Dhammameghena vassante, sabbe hontu anāsavā; yettha pacchimakā sattā, sotāpannā bhavantu te.* (धम्ममेघेन वस्सन्ते, सब्बे होन्तु अनासवा। येत्थ पच्छिमका सत्ता, सोतापन्ना भवन्तु ते ॥) (Buddha-apadāna बुद्ध-अपदान)

attain full enlightenment (after passing through no more than seven rounds of re-birth). Evidently, having reached this high stage after getting freed from the covering defilements, what remains yet to be known by such a person would naturally amount to very little. Patanjali also links his *dharmamegha samādhi* (धर्ममेघ समाधि) with cessation of hindrances, freedom from covering defilements and there being very little requirement of further knowledge.

There is a possibility that the word *'dhammamegha'* (धम्ममेघ) with all its characteristics as met with in the Buddha's lore caught the fancy of Patanjali who gave this name to the highest *samādhi* recommended by him. To our knowledge, the word *dharmamegha* (धर्ममेघ) is not met with in Vedic or post-Vedic literature, save the Buddha's lore in its Pali form.

Like *'dharmamegha'* (धर्ममेघ), the word *'prasaṅkhyāna'* (प्रसङ्ख्यान) also has its connection with the term *'saṅkhata'* (सङ्खत) used by the Buddha in his teachings. According to him, a person who is in any of the eight jhānic states, is still in the sensory field (*saṅkhata*). There are meditators who, on attaining the higher jhānic states, become complacent so far as using the discriminative knowledge (*vivekakhyāti*) (विवेकख्याति) is concerned, thinking that they have reached the final goal while they still remain in the sensory field of mind and matter (*saṅkhata*) (सङ्खत).[1] One who keeps on working with

1. *"So evaṃ pajānāti – 'imaṃ ce ahaṃ upekkhaṃ evaṃ parisuddhaṃ evaṃ pariyodātaṃ ākāsānañcāyatanaṃ upasaṃhareyyaṃ, tadanudhammaṃ ca cittaṃ bhāveyyaṃ; saṅkhatametaṃ. Imañce ahaṃ upekkhaṃ evaṃ parisuddhaṃ evaṃ pariyodātaṃ viññāṇañcāyatanaṃ upasaṃhareyyaṃ, tadanudhammaṃ ca cittaṃ bhāveyyaṃ; saṅkhatametaṃ. Imaṃ ce ahaṃ upekkhaṃ evaṃ parisuddhaṃ evaṃ pariyodātaṃ ākiñcaññāyatanaṃ upasaṃhareyyaṃ, tadanudhammaṃ ca cittaṃ bhāveyyaṃ; saṅkhatametaṃ. Imaṃ ce ahaṃ upekkhaṃ evaṃ parisuddhaṃ evaṃ pariyodātaṃ nevasaññānāsaññāyatanaṃ upasaṃhareyyaṃ, tadanudhammaṃ ca cittaṃ bhāveyyaṃ; saṅkhatametaṃ' ti.* (Majjhima – Uparipaṇṇāsakaṃ. 40.2.19)

discriminative knowledge even in these states will experience the highest samādhi called *dharmamegha* (धर्ममेघ).

("सो एवं पजानाति - इमं चे अहं उपेक्खं एवं परिसुद्धं एवं परियोदातं आकासानञ्चायतनं उपसंहरेय्यं, तदनुधम्मं च चित्तं भावेय्यं; सङ्खतमेतं। इमं चे अहं उपेक्खं एवं परिसुद्धं एवं परियोदातं विञ्ञाणञ्चायतनं उपसंहरेय्यं, तदनुधम्मं च चित्तं भावेय्यं; सङ्खतमेतं। इमं चे अहं उपेक्खं एवं परिसुद्धं एवं परियोदातं आकिञ्चञ्ञायतनं उपसंहरेय्यं, तदनुधम्मं च चित्तं भावेय्यं; सङ्खतमेतं। इमं चे अहं उपेक्खं एवं परिसुद्धं एवं परियोदातं नेवसञ्ञानासञ्ञायतनं उपसंहरेय्यं, तदनुधम्मं च चित्तं भावेय्यं; सङ्खतमेतं' ति। (मज्झिम० । उपरिपण्णासकं। 40.2.19)

'*Saṅkhata*' ('सङ्खत') stands for the field of mind and matter (or, in other words, the sensory field). In this field, things (including conceptions) spring into existence, continue to exist for a period and ultimately get annihilated. The property of '*saṅkhata*' (सङ्खत) is production, decay and change. The opposite of *saṅkhata* (सङ्खत) is '*a-saṅkhata*' (असङ्खत), which signifies the unconditioned or immaterial element or principle. This is an epithet of *nibbāna* (निब्बान) (which is unmade, unaggregated and immaterial). *Saṅkhatāsaṅkhatadhammā* (सङ्खतासङ्खतधम्मा) include every possible conception of the human mind. The teaching of the Buddha takes one from the *saṅkhata* (सङ्खत) field to the *a-saṅkhata* (असङ्खत) one. The means employed for this is the free play of the 'discriminative knowledge' (*vivekakhyāti* विवेकख्याति or *vipassanā* विपस्सना).

For the characteristics of *saṅkhata* (सङ्खत), refer Aṅguttara अङ्गुत्तर० (3.5.7).

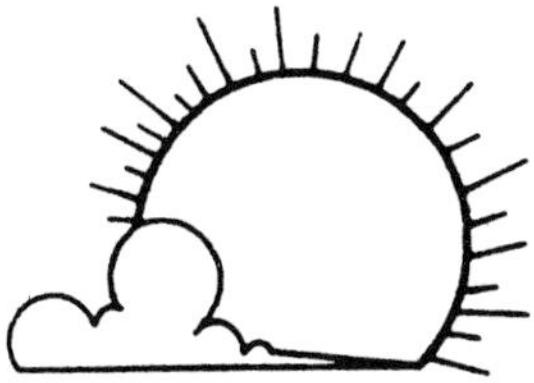

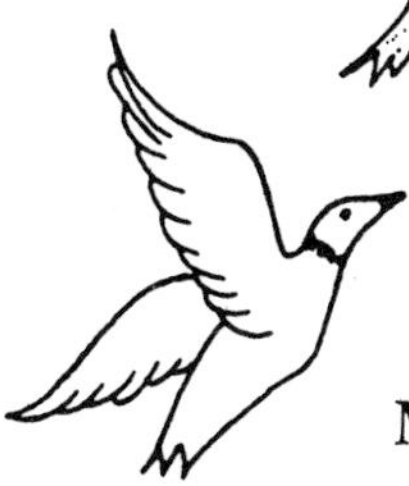

SECTION – I

(Contd.)

MATTERS CONSISTENT WITH THE BUDDHA'S TEACHING

B. TERMINOLOGICAL

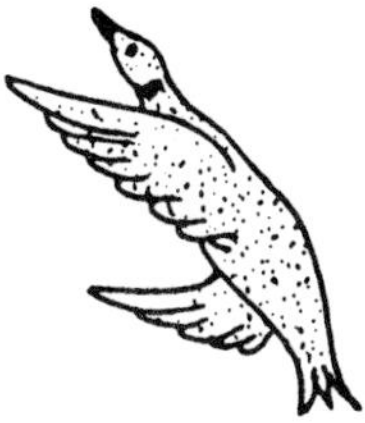

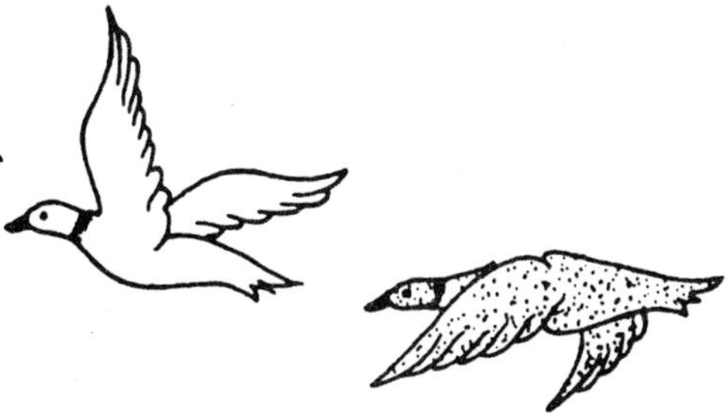

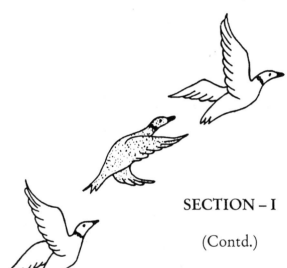

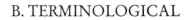

- *Adhyātmaprasādaḥ* (**अध्यात्मप्रसादः**) **(Inner quietude) –**

Patanjali employs the term *Adhyātmaprasādaḥ* (अध्यात्मप्रसादः) to express inner quietude.[1]

The Buddha used the word *ajjhattasampasādo* (अज्झत्तसम्पसादो) with the same connotation.[2]

- *Adhvan* (**अध्वन्**) **(time-path) –**

The Pali texts speak of the three bases of discourse, which are concerned with the past, future and the present (*tayo addhā*) (तयो अद्धा).[3] These are generally represented by the expression *atīto addhā, anāgato addhā, paccuppanno addhā* (अतीतो अद्धा, अनागतो अद्धा, पच्चुप्पन्नो अद्धा).

The Yoga-Sutras also employ the expressions *atīta adhva* (अतीत अध्व) and *anāgata adhva* (अनागत अध्व) to denote the past and the future stages of an entity.[4] The Yoga-bhāṣya speaks of all the three, including the present stage: *tryadhvānaḥ* (त्र्यध्वानः).[5]

---

1. *Nirvicāravaiśāradye' dhyātmaprasādaḥ* (निर्विचारवैशारद्येऽध्यात्मप्रसादः ॥) (Y.S. I.47)
2. *Ajjhattasampasādo ca pīti ca sukhaṃ ca cittekaggatā ca.* (अज्झत्तसम्पसादो च पीति च सुखं च चित्तेकग्गता च० ।) (*Majjhima. Upari-paṇṇāsakaṃ* मज्झिम० । उपरिपण्णासकं 11.1.2)
3. *"Tayome, bhikkhave, addhā. Katame tayo? Atīto addhā, anāgato addhā, paccuppanno addhā - ime kho, bhikkhave, tayo addhā" ti.* ("तयोमे, भिक्खवे, अद्धा। कतमे तयो? अतीतो अद्धा, अनागतो अद्धा, पच्चुप्पन्नो अद्धा - इमे खो, भिक्खवे, तयो अद्धा" ति ।) (*Itivuttaka* इतिवुत्तक – 3.14.14)
4. *Atītānāgataṃ svarūpato' styadhvabhedāddharmāṇām* (अतीतानागतं स्वरूपतोऽस्त्यध्वभेदाद्धर्माणाम् ॥) (Y.S. IV.12)
5. *Te khalvamī tryadhvāno dharmā vartamānā vyaktātmāno' tītānāgatāḥ sūkṣmātmānaḥ ṣaḍviśeṣarūpāḥ.*

- *Abhiniveśaḥ* (**अभिनिवेशः**) **(Clinging to one's own life, one's own existence) –**

In the Yoga-Sutras the term *abhiniveśaḥ* (अभिनिवेशः) has been used in the sense of clinging to one's own life, one's own existence.[1]

In this context, in the Pali Canon two types of clingings have been mentioned: (1) clinging to one's own eternal existence, and (2) craving to be rid of one's existence, resulting in one's total annihilation. These clingings arise because of wrong views. People in the first category wish to perpetuate life eternally, since they do not relish the idea of ceasing to be after death, while the second group feels disgusted with the cycle of worldly existences and wishes to get rid of it forever. These wrong views are called "*bhavadiṭṭhi*" (भवदिट्ठि) and '*vibhavadiṭṭhi*' (विभवदिट्ठि), respectively.[2]

- *Asampramoṣaḥ* (**असम्प्रमोषः**) **(unimpairedness, absence of loss) –**

In the Yoga-Sutras the word *asampramoṣaḥ* (असम्प्रमोषः) (unimpairedness, absence of loss) has been used with reference to an object being perceived (at this moment) while defining *smṛti* (स्मृति) (attention).[3]

(ते खल्वमी त्र्यध्वानो धर्मा वर्तमाना व्यक्तात्मानोऽतीतानागताः सूक्ष्मात्मानः षड्विशेषरूपाः ।) (Y.B. on Y.S. IV.13)

1. *Svarasavāhī viduṣo' pi tathārūḍho' bhiniveśaḥ.* (स्वरसवाही विदुषोऽपि तथारूढोऽभिनिवेशः ॥) (Y.S. II.9)
2. *Olīyanābhiniveso bhavaditthi. Atidhāvanābhiniveso vibhavaditthi.* (ओलीयनाभिनिवेसो भवदिट्ठि। अतिधावनाभिनिवेसो विभवदिट्ठि।) (*Paṭisambhidā.* पटिसम्भिदा० 1.2.5.76)
   Again, *Kathaṃ ca, bhikkhave, olīyanti eke? ...evaṃ kho, bhikkhave, olīyanti eke. ...kathaṃ ca, bhikkhave, atidhāvanti eke? ...evaṃ kho, bhikkhave, atidhāvanti eke.* (कथं च, भिक्खवे, ओलीयन्ति एके ?.... एवं खो, भिक्खवे, ओलीयन्ति एके । कथं च, भिक्खवे, अतिधावन्ति एके ?.... एवं खो, भिक्खवे, अतिधावन्ति एके ।) (Paṭisambhidā. पटिसम्भिदा० – 1.2.6.81-82)
3. *Anubhūtaviṣayāsampramoṣaḥ smṛtiḥ.* (अनुभूतविषयासम्प्रमोषः स्मृतिः ॥) (Y.S. I.11)

In the Buddha's exposition also, lack of forgetfulness (*asammusanatā*) (असम्मुसनता) is an essential characteristic of *sati* (सति) (Skt. *smṛti*) (स्मृति).[1] This aspect of *sati* (सति) is mentioned along with it at several places.[2] The Buddha used to lay stress that his mindfulness was un-impaired.[3]

- ***Ālambana* (आलम्बन) (Support) –**

The term *ālambana* (आलम्बन) occurs in the Yoga-Sutras to signify a 'support' or an 'object' for concentrating the mind upon.[4]

The same term is commonly used in the Buddha's teaching in its Pali form *ārammaṇa* (आरम्मण) to mean an 'object' (of consciousness or its concomitants). It is defined as *āramanti etthā ti ārammaṇaṃ* ('आरमन्ति एत्था ति आरम्मणं') (that is, this is called *ārammaṇa* (आरम्मण) because this is the sporting place for the mind.)

- **(तनूकरण) *(Tanūkaraṇa)* (Attenuation) –**

The word (तनूकरण) (*Tanūkaraṇa*) has been used in the Yoga-Sutras in the sense of attenuation or lessening of

---

1. *"Tattha katamā sati? Sati...asammusanatā..."* ("तत्थ कतमा सति ? सति .... असम्मुसनता.....") (Puggala. पुग्गल० – 2.35)
2. *Satiyā asammosā te devā.* (सतिया असम्मोसा ते देवा० ।) (*Dīgha. Sīlakkhandhavaggo* दीघ० । सीलक्खन्धवग्गो । 1.3.46)
3. *"Āraddhaṃ kho pana me, brāhmaṇa, viriyaṃ ahosi asallīnaṃ, upaṭṭhitā sati asammuṭṭhā..."* ("आरद्धं खो पन मे, ब्राह्मण, विरियं अहोसि असल्लीनं, उपट्ठिता सति असम्मुट्ठा.... ।") (*Majjhima, Mūlapaṇṇāsakaṃ* मज्झिम० मूलपण्णासकं । 4.3.20)
4. *Svapnanidrājñānālambanaṃ vā.* (स्वप्ननिद्राज्ञानालम्बनं वा ॥) (Y.S. I.38)

afflictions (*Kleśa-s*) (क्लेश).[1]

It was used in the same sense in the Pali Canon.[2]

- ***Divyaṃ śrotram* (दिव्यं श्रोत्रम्) (Divine Ear) –**

The term *divyaṃ śrotraṃ* (दिव्यं श्रोत्रं) (Divine Ear) appears in the Yoga-Sutras in the sense of divine power of hearing.[3]

The same term was used in the Buddha's teaching as *dibba-sota* (दिब्ब-सोत) or ***dibba sotadhātu*** (दिब्ब सोतधातु).[4] It forms one of the six Higher Powers (*cha abhiññā*) (छ अभिञ्ञा).[5]

- ***Nimna* (निम्न) (inclined towards) and *prāgbhāra* (प्राग्भार) (proximate to) –**

The words *nimna* (निम्न) and *prāgbhāra* (प्राग्भार) meaning, respectively, 'inclined towards' and 'proximate to' occur quite close to each other in one of the Yoga-Sutras.[6]

The Pali forms of these very words (*ninna* निन्न and *pabbhāra* पब्भार) having the same connotation appear quite close to each other in Pali texts also.[7]

---

1. *Samādhibhāvanārthaḥ kleśatanūkaraṇārthaśca.* (समाधिभावनार्थः क्लेशतनूकरणार्थश्च ॥) (Y.S. II.2)
2. Vinaya II. 316 (P.T.S.)
Again, in slightly different form, but with the same connotation— "*Puna caparaṃ, Mahāli, bhikkhu tiṇṇaṃ saṃyojanānaṃ parikkhayā rāgadosamohānaṃ tanuttā sakadāgamī hoti....*" (पुन चपरं, महालि, भिक्खु तिण्णं संयोजनानं परिक्खया रागदोसमोहानं तनुत्ता सकदागामी होति....") (*Dīgha. Sīlakkhandhavaggo* दीघ. सीलक्खन्धवग्गो- 6.3.15)
3. *Śrotrākāśayoḥ sambandhasaṃyamāddivyaṃ śrotram.* (श्रोत्राकाशयोः सम्बन्धसंयमाद्दिव्यं श्रोत्रम् ॥) (Y.S. III.41)
4. *Dīgha. Silakkhandhavaggo* (दीघ० । सीलक्खन्धवग्गो) । 2.5.91
5. *Dīgha. Pāthikavaggo* (दीघ० । पाथिकवग्गो ।) 11.1.7
6. *Tadā vivekanimnaṃ kaivalyaprāgbhāraṃ cittam.* (तदा विवेकनिम्नं कैवल्यप्राग्भारं चित्तम् ॥) (Y.S. IV.26)
7. *Puna caparaṃ, khīṇāsavassa bhikkhuno vivekaninnaṃ cittaṃ hoti vivekapoṇaṃ vivekapabbhāraṃ.* (पुन चपरं खीणासवस्स भिक्खुनो

- ***Nirodha* (निरोध) (Cessation) –**

The word *nirodha* (निरोध) (cessation) has been used at several places in the Yoga-Sutras.[1]

This word was of frequent occurrence in the Buddha's expositions also with the same connotation.[2]

- ***Prajñāloka* (प्रज्ञालोक) (the light of intuitive knowledge) –**

The term *prajñāloka* (प्रज्ञालोक) (the light of intuitive knowledge) occurring in the Yoga-Sutras[3] is met with in the Tipiṭaka as *paññāloko* (पञ्ञा-लोको). Four types of light find mention therein: sun-light, moon-light, light of fire, and light of intuitive knowledge. The last one is stated to be the chief or foremost amongst all.[4]

विवेकनिन्नं चित्तं होति विवेकपोणं विवेकपब्भारं....।) (*Paṭisambhidā.* पटिसम्भिदा॰ 2.9.2.26)

1. *Yogaścittavṛttinirodhaḥ. Abhyāsavairāgyābhyāṃ tannirodhaḥ. Tasyāpi nirodhe sarvanirodhānnirbījaḥ samādhiḥ.* (योगश्चित्तवृत्तिनिरोधः॥ अभ्यासवैराग्याभ्यां तन्निरोधः॥ तस्यापि निरोधे सर्वनिरोधान्निर्बीजः समाधिः॥) (Y.S. I.2, 12, 51) *Vyutthānanirodhasaṃskārayorabhibhavaprādurbhāvau nirodhakṣaṇacittānvayo nirodhapariṇāmaḥ.* (व्युत्थाननिरोधसंस्कारयोरभिभवप्रादुर्भावौ निरोधक्षणचित्तान्वयो निरोधपरिणामः॥) (Y.S. II.9)
2. E.g., *dukkhakkhandhassa nirodho, saṅkhārānaṃ nirodho, nirodhadhammaṃ, nirodhanissitaṃ, nirodhānupassī, dukkhanirodhagāminī paṭipadā. Avijjā tveva asesa-virāga-nirodhā saṅkhāranirodho; saṅkhāranirodhā viññāṇanirodho; viññāṇanirodhā nāmarūpanirodho;* (दुक्खक्खन्धस्स निरोधो, सङ्खारानं निरोधो, निरोधधम्मं, निरोधनिस्सितं, निरोधानुपस्सी, दुक्खनिरोधगामिनी पटिपदा। अविज्जा त्वेव असेस-विराग-निरोधा सङ्खारनिरोधो; सङ्खारनिरोधा विञ्ञाणनिरोधो; विञ्ञाणनिरोधा नामरूपनिरोधो;) etc.
3. *Tajjayāt prajñālokaḥ.* (तज्जयात्प्रज्ञालोकः॥) (Y.S. III.5)
4. *"Cattārome, bhikkhave, ālokā. Katame cattāro? Candāloko, suriyāloko, aggāloko, paññāloko – 'ime kho, bhikkhave, cattāro ālokā.*

- ***Prātibha* (प्रातिभ) (analytical knowledge par excellence) –**

In the Yoga-Sutras the term *prātibha* (प्रातिभ) has been employed in two Sutras. The former states that the meditator discerns all because of his analytical knowledge. The second enumerates the various types of super-sensory powers attained as a result of such knowledge.[1]

The cognate expression used in the Buddha's teaching is *paṭibhāna* (पटिभान) which is the fourth and the last of the analytical sciences leading to perfect understanding of the various phenomena.[2]

- ***Bhāvanā* (भावना) (mental development) –**

The term *bhāvanā* (भावना) (mental development) occurs at several places in the Yoga-Sutras.[3]

Etadaggaṃ, bhikkhave, imesaṃ catunnaṃ ālokānaṃ yadidaṃ paññāloko" ti. ("चत्तारोमे, भिक्खवे, आलोका। कतमे चत्तारो? चन्दालोको, सुरियालोको, अग्गालोको, पञ्ञालोको - इमे खो, भिक्खवे, चत्तारो आलोका। एतदग्गं, भिक्खवे, इमेसं चतुन्नं आलोकानं यदिदं पञ्ञालोको" ति।) (*Aṅguttara.* अङ्गुत्तर॰ - 4.15.3.1)

1. *Prātibhādvā sarvam. Tataḥ prātibhaśrāvaṇavedanādarśāsvādavārtā jāyante.* (प्रातिभाद् वा सर्वम्॥ ततः प्रातिभश्रावणवेदनादर्शास्वादवार्ता जायन्ते॥) (Y.S. III. 32,35)
2. *The four sciences are: atthapaṭisambhidā, dhammapaṭisambhidā, niruttipaṭisambhidā and paṭibhānapaṭisambhidā* (अत्थपटिसम्भिदा, धम्मपटिसम्भिदा, निरुत्तिपटिसम्भिदा, पटिभानपटिसम्भिदा) (i.e., those relating to exposition, phenomena, intuitive knowledge of words and a wonderful ability to divide, dissect, anatomise and analyse things). (*Paṭisambhidā.* (पटिसम्भिदा॰ - 1.1.0.25-28) Sāriputta, the eminent disciple of the Buddha, claimed to possess all these. (*Aṅguttara.* अङ्गुत्तर॰ - 4.18.2)
3. *Tajjapastadarthabhāvanaṃ. Maitrīkaruṇāmuditopekṣāṇāṃ . . . bhāvanātaścittaprasādanaṃ.* (तज्जपस्तदर्थभावनम्॥ मैत्रीकरुणामुदितोपेक्षाणां .... भावनातश्चित्तप्रसादनम्॥) (Y.S. I.28,33)

This very term is met with frequently in the Buddha's lore, e.g., *lokiyā bhāvanā, lokuttarā bhāvanā, indriyabhāvanā, samatha bhāvanā, vipassanā bhāvanā* (लोकिया भावना, लोकुत्तरा भावना, इन्द्रियभावना, समथ भावना, विपस्सना भावना), etc. It also signifies a Right Effort under *sammā vāyāmo* (सम्मा वायामो).[1] Different types of *bhāvanā* (भावना) stand enumerated under the heading *'bhāvanānaṃ bhedā'* ('भावनानं भेदा') in a Pali text.[2]

• *Bhūmi* (भूमि) (Plane) –

The word *bhūmi* (भूमि) occurs in the Yoga-Sutras in the sense of a 'plane'.[3]

This word was used in the Buddha's expositions in the same sense. The four planes recognised by him are the sensual-desire sphere, the material sphere, the immaterial sphere, and the unincluded sphere.[4]

Samādhibhāvanārthaḥ kleśatanūkaraṇārthaśca. (समाधिभावनार्थ: क्लेशतनूकरणार्थश्च ॥) (Y.S. II.2)
Viśeṣadarśina ātmabhāvabhāvanāvinivṛttiḥ. (विशेषदर्शिन आत्मभावभावनाविनिवृत्ति: ॥) (Y.S. IV. 25)

1. *"Saṃvaro ca pahānaṃ ca, bhāvanā anurakkhaṇā.*
Ete padhānā cattāro, desitādiccabandhunā.
Yehi bhikkhu idhātāpī, khayaṃ dukkhassa pāpuṇe" ti.
("संवरो च पहानं च, भावना अनुरक्खणा।
एते पधाना चत्तारो, देसितादिच्चबन्धुना।
येहि भिक्खु इधातापी, खयं दुक्खस्स पापुणे" ति)
(*Aṅguttara.* अङ्गुत्तर० - 4.2.4)
2. *Paṭisambhidā* पटिसम्भिदा० - 1.1.1.72-75
3. *Tasya bhūmiṣu viniyogaḥ.* (तस्य भूमिषु विनियोग: ॥) (Y.S. III.6)
4. *Catasso bhūmiyo — kāmāvacarā bhūmi, rūpāvacarā bhūmi, arūpāvacarā bhūmi, apariyāpannā bhūmi.* (चतस्सो भूमियो -- कामावचरा भूमि, रूपावचरा भूमि, अरूपावचरा भूमि, अपरियापन्ना भूमि।) (*Paṭisambhidā* पटिसम्भिदा० - 1.1.18.182)

- ***Mṛdu-madhya-adhimātra* (मृदु - मध्य - अधिमात्र) (mild, moderate, intense) –**

The expression *mṛdu-madhya-adhimātra* (मृदु - मध्य - अधिमात्र) (mild, moderate, intense) used in the Yoga-Sutras[1] found usage in the Buddha's exposition also, with the only difference that the word *adhimātra* (अधिमात्र) figured as the Pali equivalent of the Sanskrit word *tīkṣṇa* (तीक्ष्ण) (both having almost the same meaning.) Example: "*tikhinindriyo majjhimindriyo mudindriyo*" ("तिखिनिन्द्रियो मज्झिमिन्द्रियो मुदिन्द्रियो") (i.e., having acute senses, having ordinary senses, having dull senses.)[2]

- ***Yogī* (योगी) (a. a follower of the Yoga-System; b. one given to contemplation) –**

The term *yogī* (योगी) appears in the Yoga-Sutras to mean a follower of the Yoga-System or one given to contemplation.[3]

The expression used in the Pali texts is *yogāvacara* (योगावचर)[4]. In the Visuddhimagga this is the usual term for the disciple cultivating mental concentration.

- ***Vaśīkāra* (वशीकार) (mastery) –**

The term *vaśīkāra* (वशीकार) has been used in the

---

1. *Mṛdumadhyādhimātratvāttato' pi viśeṣaḥ.* (मृदुमध्याधिमात्रत्वात्ततोऽपि विशेषः ॥) (Y.S. I.22)
2. Another illustration: "*paññavā puggalo tikkhindriyo, duppañño puggalo mudindriyo.*" ("पञ्ञवा पुग्गलो तिक्खिन्द्रियो, दुप्पञ्ञो पुग्गलो मुदिन्द्रियो।") Paṭisambhidā पटिसम्भिदा॰ - 1.4.5.21.83
3. *Karmāśuklākṛṣṇaṃ Yoginastrividhamitareṣāṃ.* (कर्माशुक्लाकृष्णं योगिनस्त्रिविधमितरेषाम् ॥) (Y.S. III.7)
4. *Yogāvacaro pañcindriyāni avikkhepe patiṭṭhāpeti,* ...(योगावचरो पञ्चिन्द्रियानि अविक्खेपे पतिट्ठापेति,.... ।) (*Paṭisambhidā.* पटिसम्भिदा॰- 1.4.4.17.62)

Yoga-Sutras in the sense of 'mastery'.[1]

The word *vasī* (वसी) (Skt. *vaśī*) (वशी) was in common use in the Buddha's expositions. Sāriputta had, for instance, attained mastery (*vasippatto*) (वसिप्पत्तो) in Noble Conduct, Noble Concentration, Noble Wisdom and Noble Salvation.[2] Mastery over sense-organs was expressed as *indriyānaṃ vasībhāvatā* (इन्द्रियानं वसीभावता).[3] Elders used to proclaim that they had attained mastery in *samādhi-s*[4], supernormal powers,[5] etc. In a certain text five kinds of masteries have been mentioned: mastery in adverting, attaining, resolving, emerging and reviewing.[6]

- ***Vitarka* (वितर्क) and *vicāra* (विचार) (thought-conception and rolling in thoughts) –**

In the Yoga-Sutras the terms *vitarka* (वितर्क) and *vicāra* (विचार) signify 'initial application of mind to the object' and

---

1. *Paramāṇuparamamamahatvānto' sya vaśīkāraḥ.* (परमाणुपरममहत्त्वान्तोऽस्य वशीकार: ॥) (Y.S. I.40)
2. "*Yaṃ kho taṃ, bhikkhave…, Sāriputtameva taṃ sammā vadamāno vadeyya…'vasippatto…ariyasmiṃ sīlasmiṃ, vasippatto…samādhismiṃ, vasippatto…ariyāya paññāya, vasippatto…ariyāya vimuttiyā' ti.* ("यं खो तं, भिक्खवे… सारिपुत्तमेव तं सम्मा वदमानो वदेय्य - 'वसिप्पत्तो ….अरियस्मिं सीलस्मिं, वसिप्पत्तो….समाधिस्मिं, वसिप्पत्तो…..अरियाय पञ्ञाय, वसिप्पत्तो…..अरियाय विमुत्तिया' ति।) (*Majjhima. Uparipaṇṇāsakaṃ* मज्झिम० । उपरिपण्णासकं 11.2.5)
3. *Paṭisambhidā.* पटिसम्भिदा० – 1.1.55.267
4. E.g., *Pilindavaccha* (पिलिन्दवच्छ) proclaims: "*Vasī homi samādhisu.*" ("वसी होमि समाधिसु।") (*Therāpadāna* थेरापदान – 40.1.157)
5. *Paṭācārā* (पटाचारा) proclaims: "*Iddhīsu ca vasī homi.*" ("इद्धीसु च वसी होमि।") (*Therī apadāna* थेरीअपदान – 2.10.503)
6. *Pañca vasiyo - āvajjanavasī, samāpajjanavasī, adhiṭṭhānavasī, vuṭṭhānavasī, paccavekkhaṇāvasī* - (पञ्च वसियो। आवज्जनवसी, समापज्जनवसी, अधिट्ठानवसी, वुट्ठानवसी, पच्चवेक्खणावसी।) (*Paṭisambhidā.* पटिसम्भिदा० – 1.1.34.237)

'sustained attention to the object', respectively.[1]

The Pali forms of these terms *vitakka* (वितक्क) and *vicāra* (विचार) were used in the Buddha's expositions with the same connotation.

• *Vaiśāradya* (वैशारद्य) (matter of confidence) –

In the Yoga-Sutras the term *vaiśāradya* (वैशारद्य) is met with in the sense of 'a matter of confidence'. The relevant Sutra[2] states when the *nirvicāra samādhi* (निर्विचार समाधि) (that is, concentration without sustained attention to the object) becomes a matter of confidence, there arises inner quietude (*adhyātmaprasādaḥ*) (अध्यात्मप्रसाद:).

The term *vaiśāradya* (वैशारद्य), referred to above, seems to allude to the Pali term *vesārajja* (वेसारज्ज). An enlightened person (*Tathāgata*) (तथागत) is reputed to have four *vesārajja-s* (वेसारज्ज) or subjects of confidence.[3] An *ariyapuggala* (अरियपुग्गल), still under training in Dhamma, had to imbibe five qualities to develop confidence in him.[4]

---

1. *Vitarkavicārānandāsmitārūpānugamātsamprajñātaḥ.* (वितर्कविचारानन्दास्मितारूपानुगमात्सम्प्रज्ञात: ॥) (Y.S. I.17)
2. *Nirvicāravaiśāradye' dhyātmaprasādaḥ.* (निर्विचार-वैशारद्येऽध्यात्मप्रसाद: ॥) (Y.S. I.47)
3. "*Cattārimāni, bhikkhave, tathāgatassa vesārajjāni...*" (चत्तारिमानि, भिक्खवे, तथागतस्स वेसारज्जानि....") (*Aṅguttara.* अङ्गुत्तर० - 4.1.8)
4. *Pañcime, bhikkhave, sekhavesārajjakaraṇā dhammā. Katame pañca? Idha, bhikkhave, bhikkhu saddho hoti, sīlavā hoti, bahussuto hoti, āraddhaviriyo hoti, paññavā hoti.* ('पञ्चिमे, भिक्खवे, सेखवेसारज्जकरणा धम्मा। कतमे पञ्च ? इध, भिक्खवे, भिक्खु सद्धो होति, सीलवा होति, बहुस्सुतो होति, आरद्धविरियो होति, पञ्ञवा होति'।) (*Aṅguttara.* अङ्गुत्तर० - 5.11.1.1)

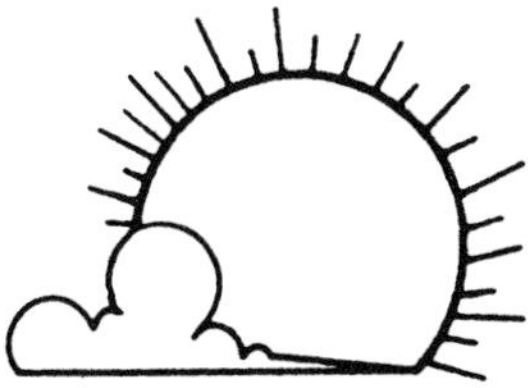

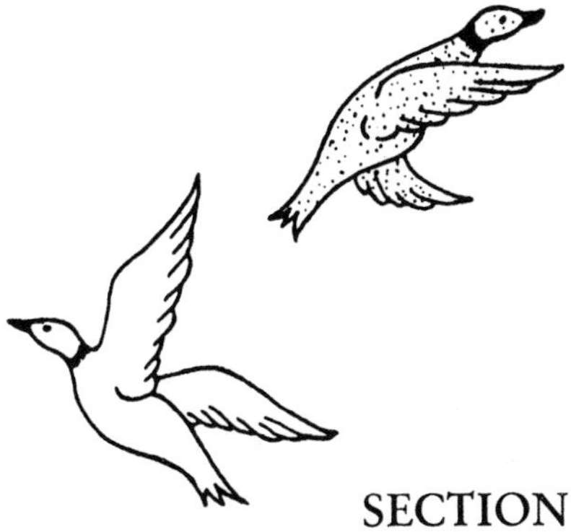

SECTION – II

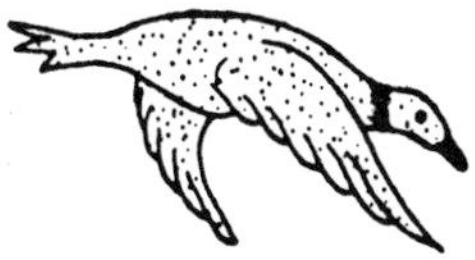

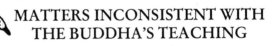

MATTERS INCONSISTENT WITH THE BUDDHA'S TEACHING

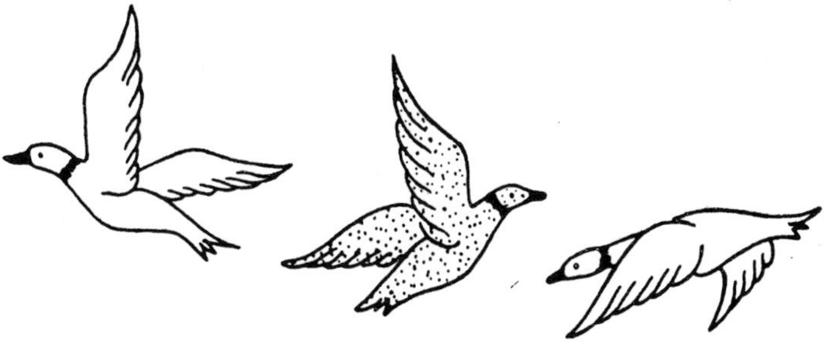

• The Aim –

According to Patanjali, the aim of Yoga is the cessation of mental fluctuations (*cittavṛttinirodhaḥ*) (चित्तवृत्तिनिरोधः).[1]

According to the Buddha, the aim of meditation is to experience the cessation of the mind itself (*cittanirodha*) (चित्तनिरोध).[2]

• Scriptural authority as a means of valid knowledge–

For Patanjali perception (*pratyakṣa*) (प्रत्यक्ष), inference (*anumāna*) (अनुमान) and scriptural authority (*āgama*) (आगम) formed the means of valid knowledge.[3]

The Buddha did not accept scriptural authority as a means of valid knowledge. The Pali Canon presents a list of six kinds of authorities which the Buddha has criticised.[4] They are as follows:

1. *anussava* (अनुस्सव) (the Vedic tradition)
2. *paramparā* (परम्परा) (tradition in general)
3. *iti kirā* (report or hearsay)
4. *piṭaka-sampadā* (पिटक-सम्पदा) (scripture in general)
5. *bhavyarūpyatā* (भव्यरूप्यता) (eminence of the speaker)
6. *samaṇo no garu* (समणो नो गरु) (prestige of the speaker)

---

1. *Yogaścittavṛttinirodhaḥ* (योगश्चित्तवृत्तिनिरोधः ॥) (Y.S. I.2)
2. This is also called 'cessation of perception and sensations' (*saññā-vedayita-nirodha*) (सञ्ञा-वेदयित-निरोध). This is a higher stage as compared to *cittavṛttinirodha* (चित्तवृत्तिनिरोध).
3. *Pratyakṣānumānāgamāḥ pramāṇāni.* (प्रत्यक्षानुमानागमाः प्रमाणानि ॥) (Y.S. 1.7)
4. *Kesamutti-suttaṃ* (केसमुत्तिसुत्तं) *Aṅguttara.* अङ्गुत्तर॰ 3.7.5

• 'Self-study' (*svādhyāya*) (स्वाध्याय) as an 'Observance' (niyama) (नियम) –

Patanjali includes '*svādhyāya*' (स्वाध्याय) (self-study) amongst the five 'Observances' (*niyamāḥ*) (नियमा:) prescribed by him.[1]

The Buddha always laid stress on the actual practice of Dhamma and not merely on its theoretical aspect. An interesting account is available of a monk living in a certain forest tract. Previously he had studied a lot even during rest periods but, once having come in contact with Pure Dhamma, he laid everything aside and took to its actual practice.[2]

• Resort to verbalisation for achieving concentration of mind –

In the Yoga-Sutras it has been postulated that concentration can also be achieved through devotion to 'Lord' (*Īśvara*) (ईश्वर).[3] The word expressing the 'Lord' is the mystic syllable *Om* (ओ३म्).[4] The repetition of this word and the evocation of its meaning have to be resorted to.[5]

In the teaching of the Buddha there is no scope for verbalisation of any sort. If the aim of an aspirant is to get rid of all his mental impurities, the use of an imaginary word—howsoever sacred—can create obstacles in his way. By repeating a word or phrase one creates an artificial vibration in which one becomes engulfed. Such a vibration acts as a barrier to the observation of natural vibrations arising within the body. If one does not observe these natural vibrations, there

---

1. *Śaucasantoṣatapaḥsvādhyāyeśvarapraṇidhānāni niyamāḥ.* (शौचसन्तोषतप:स्वाध्यायेश्वरप्रणिधानानि नियमा: ॥) (Y.S. II.32)
2. *Saṃyutta.* संयुत्त० – 9.10.10
3. *Īśvarapraṇidhānād vā* (ईश्वरप्रणिधानाद्वा ॥) (Y.S. I.23)
4. *Tasya vācakaḥ praṇavaḥ.* (तस्य वाचक: प्रणव: ॥) (Y.S. I.27)
5. *Tajjapastadarthabhāvanam.* (तज्जपस्तदर्थभावनम् ॥) (Y.S. I.28)

remains no scope for getting rid of the mental impurities. Hence the precept of the Yoga-Sutras is incompatible with the Buddha's teaching.

It is, however, noteworthy that Patanjali assigns only secondary importance to the method of developing devotion towards the Lord (*Īśvarapraṇidhāna*) (ईश्वरप्रणिधान). The use of the word *vā* (वा) (or) in the Sutra suggests that this is only an alternative approach suggested by him. The method actually recommended by him seems to be the one which has been dealt with earlier, *viz.*, to practise concentration with intuitive knowledge (*samprajñāta samādhi*) (सम्प्रज्ञात समाधि) and then switch on to another (*anya*) (अन्य)[1], which takes one beyond the stage of *samprajñāna* (सम्प्रज्ञान). If this were not so, the author would have reversed the order of his recommendations, giving the first place to devotion to Lord (*Īśvarapraṇidhāna*) (ईश्वरप्रणिधान) and only the next place to the practice of concentration (*samādhi*) (समाधि).[2]

• Immutable entity called *Puruṣa* (पुरुष) –

In the Yoga-Sutras an immutable entity called *Puruṣa* (पुरुष) has been envisaged which remains aware of an individual's mental processes all the time.[3]

---

1. *Vitarkavicārānandāsmitārūpānugamāt samprajñātaḥ. Virāmapratyayābhyāsapūrvaḥ saṃskāraśeṣo' nyaḥ.* (वितर्कविचारानन्दास्मितारूपानुगमात्सम्प्रज्ञातः॥ विरामप्रत्ययाभ्यासपूर्वः संस्कारशेषोऽन्यः॥) (Y.S. I.17-18)
2. It has been mentioned in the Preface that Patanjali seems to be a codifier of what was considered to be the best in the realm of meditation in his times. It appears he included this subject-matter to satisfy a section of the population which believed in the efficacy of this approach in attaining emancipation from worldly ills. Or else, the related sutras could be interpolation of later times.
3. *Sadā jñātāścittavṛttayastatprabhoḥ puruṣasyāpariṇāmitvāt.* (सदा ज्ञाताश्चित्तवृत्तयस्तत्प्रभोः पुरुषस्यापरिणामित्वात्॥) (Y.S. IV.18)

The Buddha did not envisage any entity like *Puruṣa* (पुरुष). For him the body was *manomaya* (मनोमय), that is to say, imbued with mind.[1] The Abhidhamma texts present a detailed account of the functioning of the mind *(citta)* (चित्त) and its concomitants (*cetasika-s*) (चेतसिक).

• Arising and passing away of phenomena –

In the Yoga-Sutras one comes across use of the words "*abhibhavaprādurbhāvau*"[2] (अभिभवप्रादुर्भावौ) (dissolution and evolution), "*kṣayodayau*"[3] (क्षयोदयौ) (fall and rise) and "*śāntoditau*"[4] (शान्तोदितौ) (disappearance and appearance). These terms seem to signify the 'passing away and arising' of certain phenomena but these are not compatible with the Buddha's exposition which links the arising and passing away (*udaya-vyaya*) (उदय-व्यय) of all mind-matter phenomena with sensations (*vedanā*) (वेदना). According to him, it is in these *vedanā-s* that all mental states have their confluence[5] and it is through these alone that one actually experiences all phenomena. Patanjali is silent on this aspect—that sensations are aids to the interpretation of phenomena—and, in actual

---

1. *'Manomayesu kāyesu sabbattha pāramiṃ gato'* ('मनोमयेसु कायेसु सब्बत्थ पारमिं गतो') (*Therāpadāna* (थेरापदान) 2.4.53)
   Also see *Majjhima. Upari-paṇṇāsakaṃ* मज्झिम० । उपरिपण्णासकं । 16.3.4.
2. *Vyutthānanirodhasaṃskārayorabhibhavaprādurbhāvau nirodhakṣaṇacittānvayo nirodhapariṇāmaḥ.* (व्युत्थाननिरोधसंस्कारयोरभिभवप्रादुर्भावौ निरोधक्षणचित्तान्वयो निरोधपरिणामः ॥) (Y.S. III.9)
3. *Sarvārthataikāgratayoḥ kṣayodayau cittasya samādhipariṇāmaḥ.* (सर्वार्थतैकाग्रतयोः क्षयोदयौ चित्तस्य समाधिपरिणामः ॥) (Y.S. III.19)
4. *Tataḥ punaḥ śāntoditau tulyapratyayau cittasyaikāgratāpariṇāmaḥ.* (ततः पुनः शान्तोदितौ तुल्यप्रत्ययौ चित्तस्यैकाग्रतापरिणामः ॥) (Y.S. III.12)
5. *Vedanāsamosaraṇā sabbe dhammā.* (वेदनासमोसरणा सब्बे धम्मा ।) (*Aṅguttara.* अङ्गुत्तर० 10.6.8.2)

fact, this constitutes a basic difference in the teachings of the two teachers.

The Buddha states unequivocally that the Four Noble Truths, which form the essence of his teaching, can be understood, realized and practised only through the experience of sensations (*vedanā-s*) (वेदना).[1]

According to him, it is better to spend a day witnessing the arising and passing away of phenomena than to live a life of hundred years remaining oblivious of this.[2]

• Incompatibility of terms drawn from the Sāṃkhya doctrines –

The Yoga-Sutras make use of certain terms drawn from the Sāṃkhya System of Indian Philosophy, e.g., *guṇa-s, prakṛti, pradhāna, puruṣa, liṅga, aliṅga* (गुण, प्रकृति, प्रधान, पुरुष, लिङ्ग, अलिङ्ग), etc. These terms do not have any connection with the Buddha's teaching. If, at all, some of these terms are found used in the Pali texts, their usage is not in line with the Sāṃkhyas.

• Use of '*saṃyama*' (संयम) as a technical term –

Patanjali uses the word '*saṃyama*' (संयम) in a technical sense, that is to say, the unification of the three practices of *dhāraṇā* (धारणा), *dhyāna* (ध्यान) and *samādhi* (समाधि) advocated

---

1. *Vediyamānassa kho panāhaṃ, bhikkhave, idaṃ dukkhaṃ ti paññāpemi, ayaṃ dukkha-samudayo ti paññāpemi, ayaṃ dukkha-nirodho ti paññāpemi, ayaṃ dukkha-nirodha-gāminī paṭipadā ti paññāpemi.*
(वेदियमानस्स खो पनाहं, भिक्खवे, इदं दुक्खं ति पञ्ञापेमि, अयं दुक्खसमुदयो ति पञ्ञापेमि, अयं दुक्खनिरोधो ति पञ्ञापेमि, अयं दुक्खनिरोधगामिनी पटिपदा ति पञ्ञापेमि।) (*Aṅguttara.* अङ्गुत्तर० 3.7.1)
2. *Yo ca vassasataṃ jīve, apassaṃ udayabbayam; ekāhaṃ jīvitaṃ seyyo, passato udayabbayaṃ.* (यो च वस्ससतं जीवे, अपस्सं उदयब्बयं। एकाहं जीवितं सेय्यो, पस्सतो उदयब्बयं॥) (Dhammapada धम्मपद 8.113)

by him.[1] When perfected, this helps in attaining different types of super-normal powers.[2]

The Buddha used this word in its ordinary sense.[3]

• The state of Isolation (*kaivalya*) (कैवल्य) –

According to Patanjali, the final aim of Yoga is the attainment of Isolation (*kaivalya*) (कैवल्य). Isolation results when the qualities (*guṇa-s*) (गुण), having become devoid of the object of the *Puruṣa* (पुरुष), become latent.[4]

In the Buddha's lore the terms *kevala* and *kevalī* (केवल, केवली) (Isolated) are met with. There these refer to the pure (un-mixed) state of liberation. Thus, *kevalī* (केवली) would be one who exhibits morality, concentration of mind, liberation, knowledge and mastery of the Dhamma lore of an Arahanta.[5]

The Buddha himself was called *kevalī* (केवली).[6]

---

1. *Deśabandhaścittasya dhāraṇā.* (देशबन्धश्चित्तस्य धारणा ॥) (Y.S. III.1)
Tatra pratyayaikatānatā dhyānam (तत्र प्रत्ययैकतानता ध्यानम्) (Y.S. III.2)
Tadevārthamātranirbhāsaṃ svarūpaśūnyamiva samādhiḥ. (तदेवार्थमात्रनिर्भासं स्वरूपशून्यमिव समाधिः ॥) (Y.S. III.3)
Trayamekatra saṃyamaḥ (त्रयमेकत्र संयमः ॥) (Y. S. III. 4)
2. Y.S. III.16 (onwards).
3. *Yamhi saccaṃ ca dhammo ca, ahiṃsā saṃyamo damo; sa ve vantamalo dhīro, so thero ti pavuccati.* (यम्हि सच्चं च धम्मो च, अहिंसा संयमो दमो। स वे वन्तमलो धीरो, थेरो इति पवुच्चति ॥) (Dhammapada, धम्मपद - 19.261)
4. *Puruṣārthaśūnyānāṃ guṇānāṃ pratiprasavaḥ kaivalyaṃ.* (पुरुषार्थशून्यानां प्रतिप्रसवः कैवल्यं० ॥) (Y.S. IV.34)
5. *"Asekhena ca sīlena, asekhena samādhinā, vimuttiyā ca sampanno, ñāṇena ca tathāvidho." "Sa ve pañcaṅgasampanno, pañca aṅge vivajjayaṃ, imasmiṃ dhammavinaye, kevalī iti vuccatī" ti.* ("असेखेन च सीलेन, असेखेन समाधिना। विमुत्तिया च सम्पन्नो, ञाणेन च तथाविधो ॥ "स वे पञ्चङ्गसम्पन्नो, पञ्च अङ्गे विवज्जयं। इमस्मिं धम्मविनये, केवली इति वुच्चती" ति ॥) (Aṅguttara. अङ्गुत्तर० - 10.2.2.3)
6. *Yo dhammacakkaṃ abhibhuyya kevalī, pavattayī sabbabhūtānukampī.* (यो धम्मचक्कं अभिभुय्य केवली, पवत्तयी सब्बभूतानुकम्पी।) (*Aṅguttara.* अङ्गुत्तर० - 4.1.8)

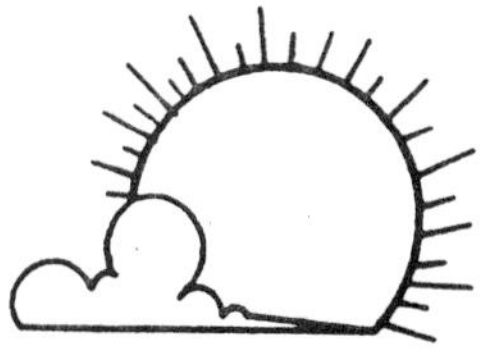

SECTION – III

SUPER-NORMAL POWERS

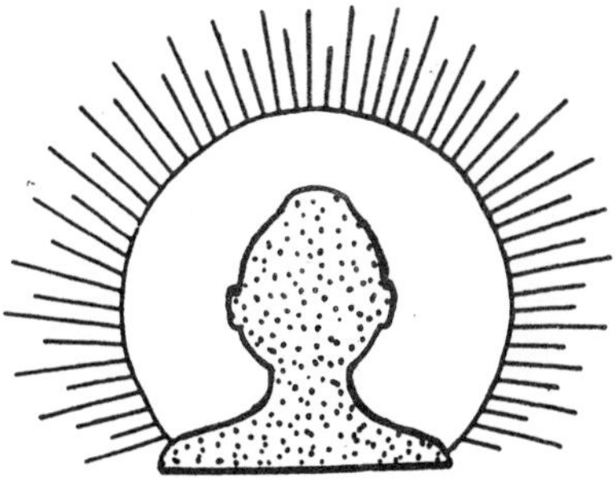

The Yoga-Sutras mention a number of super-normal powers attainable by a yogi. These include, among others, knowledge of the past and the future, knowledge of previous births, knowledge of others' mind, knowledge of the universe including arrangement and movement of stars, knowledge of the bodily system, knowledge of super-sensory perceptions, the vision of the Siddhas, power to disappear from view, power to suppress hunger and thirst, power to rove through the sky, divine power of hearing, omniscience, mind-like velocity, mastery over the elements and so on.[1]

The Buddha ordains that six Higher Powers called *cha abhiññā* (छ अभिञ्ञा) may be directly perceived.[2] These are:

(1) Mystical powers (*iddhividha*) (इद्धिविध) –

From being one, one becomes manifold, and having become manifold, one becomes one; appearing and disappearing, one passes without any obstruction through a wall, a rampart, a mountain, as if through air; one sinks into the ground and emerges from it, as if it were water; one walks on water without dividing it, as if it were solid ground; cross-legged, one roves through the sky, like a winged bird; with one's hand one touches and strokes even these—the

---

1. Y.S. III. 16-49.
2. "*Katame cha dhammā sacchikātabbā? Cha abhiññā: idhāvuso, bhikkhu anekavihitaṃ iddhividhaṃ paccanubhoti – eko pi hutvā bahudhā hoti bahudhā pi hutvā eko hoti…āsavānaṃ khayā anāsavaṃ cetovimuttiṃ paññāvimuttiṃ diṭṭheva dhamme sayaṃ abhiññā sacchikatvā upasampajja viharati.*" ("कतमे छ धम्मा सच्छिकातब्बा? छ अभिञ्ञा : इधावुसो, भिक्खु अनेकविहितं इद्धिविधं पच्चनुभोति - एको पि हुत्वा बहुधा होति बहुधा पि हुत्वा एको होति..... आसवानं खया अनासवं चेतोविमुत्तिं पञ्ञाविमुत्तिं दिट्ठेव धम्मे सयं अभिञ्ञा सच्छिकत्वा उपसम्पज्ज विहरति।") (Dīgha. *Pāthikavaggo*. दीघ० । पाथिकवग्गो। 11.1.7)

Moon and the Sun—so potent and mighty though they are; and he travels in the body as far as the Brahmā-world.

(2) Divine faculty of hearing (*dibba sotadhātu*) (दिब्ब सोतधातु) –

With a divine faculty of hearing, clear and surpassing that of human beings, one hears sounds both divine and human, whether far or near.

(3) Knowing the mind of another (*parassa cetopariyañāṇa*) (परस्स चेतोपरियञाण) –

One knows the minds of other beings, of other persons, by penetrating them with one's own mind.

(4) Recalling previous states of existence (*pubbenivāsānussati*) (पुब्बेनिवासानुस्सति) –

One calls to mind in all their modes, details and various ways one's previous states of existence.

(5) Divine vision (*dibba cakkhu*) (दिब्ब चक्खु) –

One beholds, with divine vision, clear and surpassing that of humans, beings passing away and arising, base and excellent, beautiful and ugly, gone to a happy state or gone to a woeful state, according to their deeds.

(6) Knowledge of extinction of defiling impulses (*āsavakkhayakarañāṇa*) (आसवक्खयकरञाण) –

By the destruction of the defiling impulses (*āsava-s*) (आसव), one enters on and abides in that emancipation of mind which is free from defiling impulses, having realised it by one's own super-knowledge even in one's present life.

The first five of these powers are mundane (*lokiya*) (लोकिय) as these are attainable through utmost perfection in mental concentration (*samādhi*) (समाधि), while the sixth one is super-mundane (*lokuttara*) (लोकुत्तर), attainable as it is with penetrating insight (*vipassanā*) (विपस्सना). While the other faculties might be possessed by others also, the last one can be attained only by an Enlightened Person, *i.e.*, an *arhanta* (अर्हन्त).

The Buddha and some of his distinguished disciples possessed all the six super-normal powers pre-eminently. These were so conspicuous that these could not be concealed. That is why Maha-kassapa had to proclaim that if someone were to think that he could conceal the six super-normal powers he could just as well think that an elephant, seven or seven-and-a-half cubits high, could be hidden by a tiny palm-leaf."[1]

While the actual process of attaining super-normal powers is not explained in the Yoga-Sutras (maybe, because of the *sūtra*-style which precludes lengthy treatment of subject-matter) the Buddha, at times, does explain this process.[2]

"Whenever, Ānanda, the Tathāgata concentrates body in mind and mind in body, and developing sense of ease and buoyancy abides therein, at such time, Ānanda, the body of the Tathāgata is more buoyant, more placid, more pliable, and more radiant.

"Suppose, Ānanda, a ball of iron is heated during the day. It becomes lighter, softer, more pliable, and more radiant. The same thing happens with the body of the Tathāgata.

---

1. "...*Sattaratanaṃ vā, āvuso, nāgaṃ aḍḍhaṭṭhamaratanaṃ vā tālapattikāya chādetabbaṃ maññeyya, yome cha abhiññā chādetabbaṃ maññeyyā*" *ti*.
("......सत्तरतनं वा, आवुसो, नागं अड्ढट्ठमरतनं वा तालपत्तिकाय छादेतब्बं मञ्ञेय्य, योमे छ अभिञ्ञा छादेतब्बं मञ्ञेय्या" ति) (Saṃyutta. संयुत्त॰ - 16.11.11)
2. "*Yasmiṃ, Ānanda, samaye tathāgato kāyaṃ pi citte samodahati, cittaṃ pi kāye samodahati...yāva brahmalokā pi kāyena vasaṃ vatteti...*" *ti*. ("यस्मिं, आनन्द, समये तथागतो कायं पि चित्ते समोदहति, चित्तं पि काये समोदहति....याव ब्रह्मलोका पि कायेन वसं वत्तेति।...." ति।) (*Saṃyutta.* संयुत्त॰ - 51.22.22)

"Now, Ānanda, at the time when the Tathāgata so concentrates body in mind and mind in body, His body with but little difficulty rises from the earth into the sky, and He in divers ways enjoys mystic powers, to wit: being one He becomes manifold, and so forth, and He travels in the body as far as the Brahmā world."

Accounts are available of a number of disciples of the Buddha who possessed super-normal powers in an exceptional degree. The Buddha himself named Mahāmoggallāna (महामोग्गल्लान) as the foremost among such disciples amongst the males[1] and Uppalavaṇṇā (उप्पलवण्णा) amongst the females.[2] The super-normal powers acquired by Anuruddha (अनुरुद्ध) find mention in a number of *sutta-s*.[3] The event of Sāriputta (सारिपुत्त) continuing his meditation despite a severe blow on his head from a passing demon makes interesting reading.[4]

Patanjali considers super-sensory powers as obstacles in *samādhi* but accomplishments of an exhibitive mind.[5]

---

1. *"Etadaggaṃ, bhikkhave, mama sāvakānaṃ bhikkūnaṃ iddhimantānaṃ yadidaṃ Mahāmoggallāno."* (एतदग्गं, भिक्खवे, मम सावकानं भिक्खूनं इद्धिमन्तानं यदिदं महामोग्गल्लानो।") *(Aṅguttara.* अङ्गुत्तर॰ 1.14 क. 3)
2. *"Etadaggaṃ, bhikkhave, mama sāvikānaṃ bhikkhunīnaṃ iddhimantīnaṃ yadidaṃ Uppalavaṇṇā".* ("एतदग्गं, भिक्खवे, मम साविकानं भिक्खुनीनं इद्धिमन्तीनं यदिदं उप्पलवण्णा।") (*Aṇguttara.* अङ्गुत्तर॰- 1.14 ड. 3)
3. *Saṃyutta.* संयुत्त॰-52 (Suttas, सुत्त 12-24)
4. While meditating under the open sky with a freshly shaven head, Sāriputta could stand, without much discomfort, a demon's blow which was so severe that it would, otherwise, have felled an elephant seven or seven-and-a-half cubits high, or might have split a mountain-peak (See *Udāna.* उदान॰ - 4.4.10-12)
5. *Te samādhāvupasargā vyutthāne siddhayaḥ.* (ते समाधावुपसर्गा व्युत्थाने सिद्धयः॥) (Y.S. III.37)

Vācaspati-Miśra[1] explains this as follows:

"For a man whose mind-stuff is exhibitive thinks highly of these perfections, just as a man born in misery considers even a small bit of wealth a pile of wealth. But a yogi whose mind-stuff is concentrated must avoid these (perfections) even when brought near to him. One who longs for the final goal of life, the absolute assuagement of the threefold anguish, how could he have any affection for those perfections which go counter to (the attainment) of that (goal)?"[2]

The Buddha also did not favour any obsession for super-normal powers. According to his dictum, such powers are an impediment for insight, though not for concentration, since these are obtained through concentration.[3]

The Buddha discouraged the display of super-normal powers for increasing in him the faith of the people.[4] According to him, the ability to perform miracles can be acquired by learning *Gandhārī vijjā* (गंधारी विद्या) also. It is, therefore, not proper to extol such performances. Sensing danger in them, these should rather be treated with contempt,

---

1. The author of *Tattva-vaiśāradī* (being a gloss on the Yoga-bhāṣya (योगभाष्य), the comment on Yoga-Sutras).
2. Translated by James Haughton Woods in "The Yoga-System of Patanjali" (Harvard Oriental Series-Vol. XVII).
3. *Visuddhi.* (विसुद्धि०) (III.56)
4. The Buddha was once staying at Nāḷandā in Pāvārika's mango-grove. There came to him Kevaṭṭa, a young householder, who said to him: "This Nāḷandā of ours, Sir, is rich, prosperous, populous, and full of people having faith in the Exalted One. If the Exalted One were to ask some monk to perform a miracle here, it would increase in Him the faith of the people."
   To this the Exalted One replied: "I do not, O Kevaṭṭa, teach Dhamma to *bhikkhus* that they may go to the white-robed householders to demonstrate wonders of miraculous mystic powers."*(Dīgha. Sīlakkhandhavaggo* दीघ० सीलक्खन्धवग्गो 11.1.1)

shame and disgust.[1]

One of his disciples Piṇḍola the Bhāradvāja, who possessed super-normal powers to an eminent degree, was rebuked by the Buddha for fetching down a costly bowl of sandalwood hung high up in the air by a wealthy merchant of Rājagaha on the top of a series of bamboo-poles which no other recluse or brahmin could bring down. When presented before him, he asked the monks to smash this bowl into pieces. He forbade them from exhibiting to householders works of psychic powers and, if anybody did so, he should be deemed to have committed an offence of 'wrong-doing' (*dukkaṭa*) (दुक्कट).[2]

---

1. *"Imaṃ kho ahaṃ, Kevaṭṭa, iddhipāṭihāriye ādīnavaṃ sampassamāno iddhipāṭihāriyena aṭṭīyāmi harāyāmi jigucchāmi."* ("इमं खो अहं, केवट्ट, इद्धिपाटिहारिये आदीनवं सम्पस्समानो इद्धिपाटिहारियेन अट्टीयामि हरायामि जिगुच्छामि।") (*Dīgha. Sīlakkhandhavaggo* दीघ. सीलक्खन्धवग्गो। 11.2.4)
2. *Vinaya. Cullavagga.* विनय० चुल्लवग्ग - 5.5.10

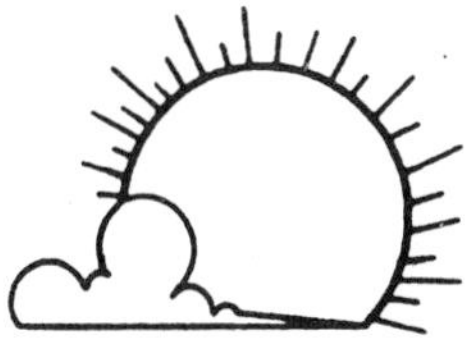

SECTION - IV

GOAL – REALISATION

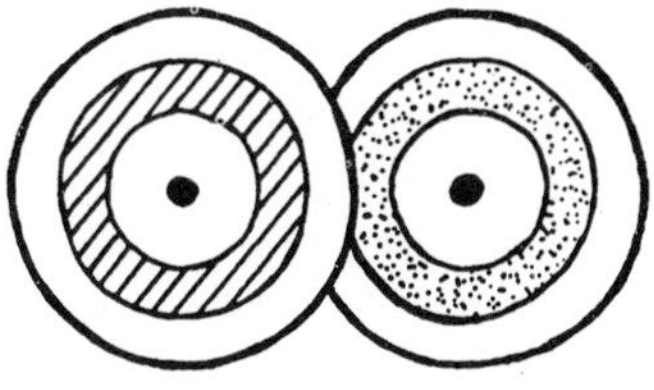

Patanjali feels that suffering which has not yet arisen should be avoided.[1] The Buddha had also ordained that effort should be made so that the unwholesome, sinful dhammas which have not yet arisen may not arise.[2] For him, suffering was a Noble Truth[3] (which could be realized at the experiential level).

According to the Yoga-Sutras, all suffering is because of the false identification of an immutable entity called *Puruṣa* (पुरुष) with the mental processes of an individual.[4] For the Buddha, the cause of all suffering lies in Desire (*taṇhā*) (तण्हा),[5] but the ultimate cause, at the deepest level is Ignorance (*avijjā*) (अविज्जा).[6]

In view of the above, the goal of Yoga is the attainment of the state of 'isolation' for the *Puruṣa* (पुरुष) which implies the

---

1. *Heyaṃ duḥkhamanāgatam* (हेयं दु:खमनागतम्) (Y.S. II.16)
2. *Anuppannānaṃ pāpakānaṃ akusalānaṃ dhammānaṃ anuppādāya ātappaṃ karaṇīyaṃ.* (अनुप्पन्नानं पापकानं अकुसलानं धम्मानं अनुप्पादाय आतप्पं करणीयं।) (Aṅguttara अङ्गुत्तर॰ - 3.5.10)
3. *Dukkhanirodhaṃ ariyasaccaṃ.* (दुक्खनिरोधं अरियसच्चं।) (*Dīgha. Pāthikavaggo* दीघ॰ । पाथिकवग्गो। 11.1.5)
4. Implied in Yoga-Sutras (I.16; III. 35, 55; IV. 18, 23, 34)
5. "*Katamaṃ cāvuso, dukkhasamudayaṃ ariyasaccaṃ ? yāyaṃ taṇhā ponobbhavikā nandīrāgasahagatā tatratatrābhinandinī, seyyathīdaṃ – kāmataṇhā bhavataṇhā vibhavataṇhā idaṃ vuccatāvuso — 'dukkhasamudayaṃ ariyasaccaṃ'.* ("कतमं चावुसो, दुक्खसमुदयं अरियसच्चं ? यायं तण्हा पोनोब्भविका नन्दीरागसहगता तत्रतत्राभिनन्दिनी, सेय्यथीदं - कामतण्हा भवतण्हा विभवतण्हा, इदं वुच्चतावुसो - 'दुक्खसमुदयं - अरियसच्चं।') *Majjhima. Upari-paṇṇāsakaṃ* मज्झिम॰ उपरिपण्णासकं। 41.2.4
6. *Avijjā* (अविज्जा) is the first link in the chain of Conditioned Arising (*paṭicca-samuppāda*) (पटिच्च-समुप्पाद). This is the root cause of all other mental impurities and hence of 'suffering'. The Buddha considered it as the worst defilement (*avijjā paramaṃ malaṃ*, अविज्जा परमं मलं) (Dhammapada, धम्मपद - 18.243)

cessation of all the mental processes of the individual. The goal of the Buddha's teaching is extinction of Desire (*taṇhā*) (तण्हा) with the eradication of Ignorance (*avijjā*) (अविज्जा). This takes place when the Ego melts away completely.

THE TWO WAYS

In order to achieve their respective goals, the aspirants of the two systems are required to proceed step-by-step as shown below.

THE YOGA-WAY –

1. The aspirant should try to adhere to the various Restraints and Observances (*yamaniyamāḥ*) (यमनियमा:)[1] prescribed in the Yoga-Sutras.
2. While sitting for meditation, he should adopt a posture which is steady and comfortable (*sthirasukha*) (स्थिरसुख).[2]
3. Then he should start the practice of *prāṇāyāma* (प्राणायाम) which would calm down the ruffled mind.[3] (Alternatively, one can have recourse to certain other objects also for stabilising the mind).[4]
4. Then he may pass through different stages of concentration which may culminate in certain attainments called *samāpatti-s* (समापत्ति) as shown below:

---

1. Yoga-Sutras (II.30,32)
2. *Sthirasukhamāsanaṃ* (स्थिरसुखमासनम्) (Y.S. II.46)
3. Yoga-Sutras (II .49, 50, 51) read with Y.S. (I.34).
4. Y.S. (I. 35, 39).

a) *Savitarkā/savicārā* (सवितर्का/सविचारा)[1] - This means *samāpatti-s* (समापत्ति) with *vitarka* (वितर्क) or *vicāra* (विचार), that is, with initial application of mind on the object or sustained attention to the object.

(b) *Nirvitarkā/nirvicārā* (निर्वितर्का/निर्विचारा)[2] - This means *samāpatti-s* (समापत्ति) without initial application of mind on the object or sustained attention to the object.

(c) In the *samāpatti* (समापत्ति) without *vicāra* (विचार) (i.e., *nirvicārā* निर्विचारा) would be produced intuitive knowledge (*prajñā*) (प्रज्ञा).[3]

(d) Intuitive knowledge (*prajñā*) (प्रज्ञा) would produce a subliminal impression (*saṃskāra*) (संस्कार) which would hinder the formation of other *saṃskāra-s* (संस्कार).[4]

(e) The restraint of the *saṃskāra-s* (संस्कार) mentioned above would result in total cessation of the mental processes[5] (enabling the aspirant to experience the

---

1. *Tatra śabdārthajñānavikalpaiḥ saṅkīrṇā savitarkā samāpattiḥ* (तत्र शब्दार्थज्ञानविकल्पैः संकीर्णा सवितर्का समापत्तिः ॥) (Y.S.I.42) *Etayaiva savicārā .. sūkṣmaviṣayā vyākhyātā* (एतयैव सविचारा..... सूक्ष्मविषया व्याख्याता ॥) (Y.S. I.44)
2. *Smṛtipariśuddhau svarūpaśūnyevārthamātranirbhāsā nirvitarkā* (स्मृतिपरिशुद्धौ स्वरूपशून्येवार्थमात्रनिर्भासा निर्वितर्का ॥) (Y.S.I.43) *Etayaiva ... nirvicārā ca sūkṣmaviṣayā vyākhyātā.* (एतयैव.... निर्विचारा च सूक्ष्मविषया व्याख्याता ॥) (Y.S. I.44)
3. *Nirvicāravaiśāradye' dhyātmaprasādaḥ. Ṛtambharā tatra prajñā.* (निर्विचारवैशारद्येऽध्यात्मप्रसादः ॥ ऋतम्भरा तत्र प्रज्ञा ॥) (Y.S.I.47,48)
4. *Tajjaḥ saṃskāro' nyasaṃskārapratibandhī* (तज्जः संस्कारोऽन्यसंस्कारप्रतिबन्धी ॥) (Y.S. I.50)
5. *Tasyāpi nirodhe sarvanirodhānnirbījaḥ samādhiḥ.* (तस्यापि निरोधे सर्वनिरोधान्निर्बीजः समाधिः ॥) (Y.S. I.51)

state of isolation of the entity called *Puruṣa* (पुरुष) from his mental processes).

THE BUDDHA-WAY –

1. The aspirant should try to observe the various Precepts on Morality (*sīla-s*) (सील) prescribed in the Buddha's teaching.[1]
2. While sitting for meditation, he should fold his legs crosswise, keep his body erect and establish mindfulness in the area around the mouth[2] (preferably, above the mouth).[3]
3. Then he should start with the mindfulness of respiration (*ānāpānassati*) (आनापानस्सति)[4] which would not only calm down his ruffled mind but would, at the same time, start purifying it.
4. The practice of *ānāpānassati* (आनापानस्सति) can lead to the experience of the following four absorptions

---

1. *Dīgha. Sīlakkhandhavaggo.* दीघ० । सीलक्खन्धवग्गो । 2.5.45.
2. *Nisīdati pallaṅkaṃ ābhujitvā, ujuṃ kāyaṃ paṇidhāya, parimukhaṃ satiṃ upaṭṭhapetvā* (निसीदति पल्लङ्कं आभुजित्वा, उजुं कायं पणिधाय, परिमुखं सतिं उपट्ठपेत्वा ।) (*Dīgha. Mahāvaggo.* दीघ० । महावग्गो । 9.2.3)
3. For this interpretation, '*parimukhaṃ*' (परिमुखं) has to be taken as '*uparimukhaṃ*' (उपरिमुखं), the initial u of *upari* (उपरि) getting elided in the same manner as *uposatha* (उपोसथ) and *udaka* (उदक) become *posatha* (पोसथ) and *daka* (दक), respectively, in Pali. This interpretation is in line with the living tradition of *ānāpānassati* (आनापानस्सति) taught by the late Sayagyi U Ba Khin of Burma and presently taught by *Kalyāṇamitta* Shri S.N. Goenka in India and round the world.
4. *Dīgha. Mahāvaggo.* दीघ० । महावग्गो । 9.2.3

(*jhāna-s*) (झान)[1] which constitute the four samāpatti-s (समापत्ति) :

(a) Ist Absorption – Detached from craving, detached from mental impurity, the aspirant enters into the first absorption, born of detachment, accompanied by initial application of mind to the object (*savitakkaṃ*) (सवितक्कं) and sustained attention to the object (*savicāraṃ*) (सविचारं) and filled with joy and bliss (*pītisukhaṃ*) (पीतिसुखं).

(b) IInd Absorption – After the subsiding of initial application of mind to the object and sustained attention to the object, by gaining inner tranquillity and oneness of mind he enters into a state free from initial application of mind to the object and sustained attention to the object (*avitakkaṃ*

---

1. *'Idha, bhikkhave, bhikkhu vivicceva kāmehi vivicca akusalehi dhammehi savitakkaṃ savicāraṃ vivekajaṃ pītisukhaṃ paṭhamaṃ jhānaṃ upasampajja viharati; vitakkavicārānaṃ vūpasamā ajjhattaṃ sampasādanaṃ cetaso ekodibhāvaṃ avitakkaṃ avicāraṃ samādhijaṃ pītisukhaṃ dutiyaṃ jhānaṃ upasampajja viharati; pītiyā ca virāgā upekkhako ca viharati sato ca sampajāno sukhaṃ ca kāyena paṭisaṃvedeti yaṃ taṃ ariyā ācikkhanti 'upekkhako satimā sukhavihārī' ti tatiyaṃ jhānaṃ upasampajja viharati; sukhassa ca pahānā dukkhassa ca pahānā pubbeva somanassadomanassānaṃ atthaṅgamā adukkhamasukhaṃ upekkhāsatipārisuddhiṃ catutthaṃ jhānaṃ upasampajja viharati.'*
('इध, भिक्खवे, भिक्खु विविच्चेव कामेहि विविच्च अकुसलेहि धम्मेहि सवितक्कं सविचारं विवेकजं पीतिसुखं पठमं झानं उपसम्पज्ज विहरति; वितक्कविचारानं वूपसमा अज्झत्तं सम्पसादनं चेतसो एकोदिभावं अवितक्कं अविचारं समाधिजं पीतिसुखं दुतियं झानं उपसम्पज्ज विहरति; पीतिया च विरागा उपेक्खको च विहरति सतो च सम्पजानो सुखं च कायेन पटिसंवेदेति यं तं अरिया आचिक्खन्ति 'उपेक्खको सतिमा सुखविहारी' ति ततियं झानं उपसम्पज्ज विहरति; सुखस्स च पहाना दुक्खस्स च पहाना पुब्बेव सोमनस्सदोमनस्सानं अत्थङ्गमा अदुक्खमसुखं उपेक्खासतिपारिसुद्धिं चतुत्थं झानं उपसम्पज्ज विहरति।') (Dīgha. Mahāvaggo दीघ० । महावग्गो। 9.5.31)

avicāraṃ) (अवितक्कं अविचारं) the second absorption, which is born of concentration and filled with joy and bliss (*samādhijaṃ pītisukhaṃ*) (समाधिजं पीतिसुखं).

(c) IIIrd Absorption – After the fading away of joy (*pītiyā ca virāgā*) (पीतिया च विरागा) he dwells in equanimity, mindfulness and constant thorough realisation of impermanence (*upekkhako ca viharati sato ca sampajāno*) (उपेक्खको च विहरति सतो च सम्पजानो), and he experiences in his body that pleasure of which the Noble Ones say 'he is equanimous, mindful, dwelling in pleasure', thus he enters the third absorption.

(d) IVth Absorption — After the eradication of bodily and mental pleasure and pain, he enters into a state beyond pleasure and pain (*adukkhaṃ asukhaṃ*) (अदुक्खं असुखं), into the fourth absorption, which is purified by equanimity and mindfulness (*upekkhāsatipārisuddhiṃ*) (उपेक्खासतिपारिसुद्धिं).

At the culmination of the IVth Absorption, one experiences a state beyond pleasure and pain (*adukkhamasukhaṃ*) (अदुक्खमसुखं), which produces a state of deep tranquillity, known as *passaddhi* (पस्सद्धि). This is a very dangerous state because it creates the illusion of the attainment of the state of *Nibbāna* and the meditator feels tempted to stop at that. When it so happens, the meditator should, with all the wisdom and patience at his command, try to go beyond this state through the experience of impermanence (*anicca*) (अनिच्च). When one succeeds in this, one attains *nirodha-samāpatti*[1] (निरोध-समापत्ति), which is another name for the state of *Nibbāna* (निब्बान).

1. Also called *saññā-vedayita-nirodha* (सञ्ञा-वेदयित-निरोध), i.e., *the cessation of perception and sensations.*

A COMPARATIVE STUDY OF THE MEDITATIVE ASPECTS

The following is a discussion on the meditative aspects of the two systems :-

- **Initial step —**

The initial step of the aspirant's adhering to a certain code of morality so as to curb unwholesome impulses of the mind is alike in both the systems.

- **Posture —**

The accent in both the systems is on the aspirant's assuming posture which can provide him or her a steady and comfortable sitting for a long time.[1] Patanjali considers such a posture can be achieved when it is effortless and the mind tends towards infinity.[2] This is precisely the Buddha's teaching, the essential ingredient of which is to let things happen as they would naturally (*yathābhūta*) (यथाभूत), that is to say, without making any effort for that. So far as the mind tending towards infinity is concerned, this takes place when all the five senses of the body stop functioning at the culmination (*samāpatti*) (समापत्ति) of the IVth Absorption, taught and practised by pre-Buddha yogis like Ālāra Kālāma and Uddaka Rāmaputta.

The Buddha stresses additionally that the aspirant should establish mindfulness around his mouth (*parimukhaṃ satiṃ*

1. Vijayā, a she-Elder, sat in her posture so comfortably that she stretched her feet on the seventh day of her meditation.
Cf. Pītisukhena ca kāyaṃ, pharitvā vihariṃ tadā. Sattamiyā pāde pasāresiṃ, tamokhandhaṃ padāliyā. (पीतिसुखेन च कायं, फरित्वा विहरिं तदा। सत्तमिया पादे पसारेसिं, तमोखन्धं पदालिया॥) (Therīgāthā थेरीगाथा-6.8.174)
2. *Prayatnaśaithilyānantyasamāpattibhyāṃ.* (प्रयत्नशैथिल्यानन्त्यसमापत्तिभ्याम्॥) (Y.S. II.47)

upaṭṭhapetvā) (परिमुखं सतिं उपट्ठपेत्वा). According to his teaching, the faculty of mindfulness (*sati*) (सति) should be made as strong as possible. It is this very faculty that keeps the other faculties on their toes, and regulates the whole process of meditation. As the salt is an absolute necessity in all curries, so is *sati* (सति) on every step of meditation.[1]

- **Practice of *prāṇāyāma* (प्राणायाम) vis-s-vis *ānāpāna* (आनापान) —**

As in the case of postures (*āsana-s*) (आसन), so also in the matter of *prāṇāyāma* (प्राणायाम) so much has been written by other writers on Yoga which Patanjali never meant.[2] Patanjali (like the Buddha) did realize that the breath had close connection with the mind and that was the reason why excitement, anger, agitation, etc. led to short and irregular breathing.[3] In order to soothe the ruffled mind of such a person, he prescribed the practice of Prāṇāyāma. He has defined it simply as the division or separation (*vichheda*) (विच्छेद) of the movements of in-breathing and out-breathing (*śvāsapraśvāsayorgativicchedaḥ*) (श्वास-प्रश्वासयो-र्गतिविच्छेद:)[4] and then he proceeds to lay down that the outward, the inward and the static conditions of breath should be perceived within a limited area (*deśa*) (देश), over a time (*kāla*) (काल) and as to its

1. *Tenāha – "Sati ca pana sabbatthikā vuttā bhagavatā. Kiṅkāraṇā ? Cittaṃ hi satipaṭisaraṇaṃ, ārakkhapaccupaṭṭhānā ca sati, na vinā satiyā cittassa paggahaniggaho hotī" ti.* (तेनाह - "सति च पन सब्बत्थिका वुत्ता भगवता। किंकारणा? चित्तं हि सतिपटिसरणं, आरक्खपच्चुपट्ठाना च सति, न विना सतिया चित्तस्स पग्गहनिग्गहो होती" ति।) (Visuddhi. विसुद्धि० 4.49)
2. *Gheraṇḍa Saṃhitā* (घेरण्ड संहिता), for example, dedicates one whole chapter with 96 stanzas to *prāṇāyāma* (प्राणायाम), but 45 stanzas only to *dhyāna* (ध्यान) and *samādhi* (समाधि).
3. *Duḥkhadaurmanasyāṅgamejayatvaśvāsapraśvāsā vikṣepasahabhuvaḥ.* (दु:खदौर्मनस्याङ्गमेजयत्वश्वासप्रश्वासा विक्षेपसहभुव: ॥) (Y.S.I.31)
4. Y.S. (II.49).

span[1] (*saṅkhyā*) (संख्या). When this is done, the depth (i.e., grossness) of breath begins to give way to shallowness (i.e., fineness) (*dīrghasūkṣmaḥ*) (दीर्घसूक्ष्म:).[2] Then he mentions a fourth stage of Prāṇāyāma which casts aside the business of external and internal (breathing).[3] In this stage, the breath seems to come to a total stop — a phenomenon popularly known as *svataḥ kumbhaka* (स्वत: कुम्भक).

In the Yoga-Sutras we do not come across any sutra wherein its author seems to advocate retention of breath with effort, as is being practised these days in the name of *Pātañjala Yoga* (पातञ्जल योग). This is a practice of the Haṭhayoga (हठयोग)[4] which has no connection with the *Pātañjala Yoga* (पातञ्जल योग). For Patanjali, *prāṇāyāma* (प्राणायाम) is nothing but the stretch of Prāṇa (*prāṇa* + *āyāma*) (प्राण+आयाम), either when it goes in (*śvāsa*) (श्वास) or when it comes out (*praśvāsa*) (प्रश्वास). Its flow makes us aware of its three stages, viz., external, internal and static. This is perceived in its totality in all these stages (*pari-dṛṣṭaḥ*) (परि-दृष्ट:), when, gradually, from its gross stage it becomes subtler and subtler (*dīrgha-sūkṣmaḥ*) (दीर्घ-सूक्ष्म:). When this process continues unabated and the respiration becomes subtle to the extreme, one may experience the fourth

---

1. Here the word *saṅkhyā* (संख्या) is not to be interpreted in the sense of 'enumeration' but 'span'. This word seems to echo the sense of the Pali word *saṅkhata* (सङ्खत) , which stands for all countable or measurable phenomena of the mundane world. How the awareness of the 'span' of the breath (i.e., its extensiveness or brevity) results in its becoming subtler and subtler till its practitioner becomes established in equanimity is explained in one of the succeeding paragraphs.
2. *Bāhyābhyantarastambhavṛttirdeśakālasaṅkhyābhiḥ paridṛṣṭo dīrghasūkṣmaḥ*. (बाह्याभ्यन्तरस्तम्भवृत्तिर्देशकालसंख्याभि: परिदृष्टो दीर्घसूक्ष्म: ॥) (Y.S.II.50)
3. *Bāhyābhyantaraviṣayākṣepī caturthaḥ*. (बाह्याभ्यन्तरविषयाक्षेपी चतुर्थ: ॥) (Y.S. II.51)
4. *Cf.* Ernst E. Wood, *Practical Yoga—Ancient and Modern*, p.121.

stage of Prāṇāyāma where there is absolutely no movement of respiration, either external or internal.

In this respect, Pātañjala Yoga-Sutra is quite close to the Buddha's teaching. The latter also does not advocate any meddling with the natural flow of respiration. It recommends only its observation in its natural course which, gradually, results in the deep (gross) breath becoming shorter and shorter (subtler and subtler) till a stage is reached when one experiences stoppage of respiration (*kumbhaka*) (कुम्भक) for different durations.[1] This stoppage, however, is natural and automatic and not at all a forced or attempted retention of breath as prescribed in the *haṭhayoga* (हठयोग).

The practice of *ānāpānassati* (आनापानस्सति) (mindfulness on in-breathing and out-breathing) as recommended by the

---

1. There is complete stoppage of respiration when the state of *saññāvedayitanirodha* (सञ्ञावेदयितनिरोध) (cessation of perception and sensations) is attained. Dhammadinnā, an Enlightened Nun, explained to Visākha, a meditator, when the state of *saññāvedayitanirodha* is attained, activity of speech is stopped first, then activity of the body, and lastly activity of the mind. She further explained that 'activity of speech' is initial application of mind to an object and its sustained attention to that object; 'activity of body' is in-breaths and out-breaths; and 'activity of mind' is perception and sensations. She also gave reasons as to why these three types of activities have to be understood in this manner.
   Cf. Tayo me, āvuso Visākha, saṅkhārā – kāyasaṅkhāro, vacīsaṅkhāro, cittasaṅkhāro.... Assāsapassāsā kho, āvuso Visākha, kāyasaṅkhāro, vitakkavicārā vacīsaṅkhāro, saññā ca vedanā ca cittasaṇkhāro .... Saññāvedayitanirodhaṃ samāpajjantassa kho, āvuso Visākha, bhikkhuno paṭhamaṃ nirujjhati vacīsaṅkhāro, tato kāyasaṅkhāro, tato cittasaṅkhāro. (तयो मे, आवुसो विसाख, सङ्खारा - कायसङ्खारो, वचीसङ्खारो, चित्तसङ्खारो।..... अस्सासपस्सासा खो, आवुसो विसाख, कायसङ्खारो, वितक्कविचारा वचीसङ्खारो, सञ्ञा च वेदना च चित्तसङ्खारो। सञ्ञावेदयितनिरोधं समापज्जन्तस्स खो, आवुसो विसाख, भिक्खुनो पठमं निरुज्झति वचीसङ्खारो, ततो कायसङ्खारो, ततो चित्तसङ्खारो।) (Majjhima Mūlapaṇṇāsakaṃ मज्झिम० । मूलपण्णासकं। 44.3.5/6)

Buddha is one of the most important exercises for reaching mental concentration and the four Absorptions (*jhāna-s*) (झान). Its detailed description is given in *Paṭisambhidāmaggo* (पटिसम्भिदामग्गो) (a Pali text) under the caption *Ānāpānassatikatha* (आनापानस्सतिकथा). It has been mentioned therein that the aspirant breathes in a long in-breath reckoned by extent (*addhāna-saṅkhāte*) (अद्धानसङ्खाते). He breathes out a long out-breath reckoned by extent. He breathes in and breathes out long in-breaths and long out-breaths reckoned by extent. By doing so, zeal (*chanda*) (छन्द) arises and the breath becomes subtler than before. By continuing this process, gladness (*pāmojja*) (पामोज्ज) arises and the breath becomes subtler still. By still continuing the process, the mind turns away from the long in-breaths and out-breaths, and equanimity (*upekkhā*) (उपेक्खा) is established.[1] In the case of in-breaths and out-breaths being short, these are reckoned by brevity (*ittara-saṅkhāte*) (इत्तरसङ्खाते). Here also, by continuing the process, arise gradually zeal and gladness, and the mind turning away from short in-breaths and out-breaths, equanimity is established.[2] The words *addhāna-saṅkhāte* (अद्धानसङ्खाते) and *ittara-saṅkhāte* (इत्तरसङ्खाते), alluding to the 'span' of breath (whether by way of extensiveness or brevity) are of great significance since these seem to provide the key to the true

---

1. *Dīghaṃ assāsaṃ addhānasaṅkhāte assasati, dīghaṃ passāsaṃ addhānasaṅkhāte passasati, dīghaṃ assāsapassāsaṃ addhānasaṅkhāte assasati pi passasati pi .... upekkhā saṇṭhāti.* (दीघं अस्सासं अद्धानसङ्खाते अस्ससति, दीघं पस्सासं अद्धानसङ्खाते पस्ससति, दीघं अस्सासपस्सासं अद्धानसङ्खाते अस्ससति पि पस्ससति पि। .....उपेक्खा सण्ठाति।) (Paṭisambhidā पटिसम्भिदा॰ - 1.3.4.32)
2. *Rassaṃ assāsaṃ ittarasaṅkhāte assasati, rassaṃ passāsaṃ ittarasaṅkhāte passasati, rassaṃ assāsapassāsaṃ ittarasaṅkhāte assasati pi passasati pi ... upekkhā saṇṭhāti.* (रस्सं अस्सासं इत्तरसङ्खाते अस्ससति, रस्सं पस्सासं इत्तरसङ्खाते पस्ससति, रस्सं अस्सासपस्सासं इत्तरसङ्खाते अस्ससति पि पस्ससति पि। ...उपेक्खा सण्ठाति।) (Paṭisambhidā. पटिसम्भिदा॰–1.3.4.52).

interpretation of the word *saṅkhyā* (संख्या) in Patanjali's Yoga-Sutra (II. 50)

• Subject of meditation –

Patanjali mentions a few subjects of meditation for stabilizing the mind and ends up by saying that an aspirant may, alternatively, meditate on some object of his choice : *yathābhimatadhyānād vā* (यथाभिमतध्यानाद् वा).[1] He also recommends the repetition of the mystic syllable *Om* (ओ३म्) with the evocation of its meaning.[2]

In the Buddha's exposition forty subjects of meditation have been enumerated, one of these being the mindfulness of respiration (*ānāpānassati*) (आनापानस्सति).[3] This subject of meditation is considered to be highly beneficial because, in the words of the Buddha, 'when developed and much practised, it perfects the fourfold establishing of mindfulness (*satipaṭṭhāna*) (सतिपट्ठान). The fourfold establishing of mindfulness, when developed and much practised, perfects the seven factors of enlightenment (*bojjhaṅga-s*) (बोज्झङ्ग). The seven factors of enlightenment, when developed and much practised, perfect deliverance by wisdom (*vijjāvimutti*) (विज्जाविमुत्ति)'[4] A

---

1. Y.S.(I. 35-39).
2. Y.S.(I. 27-28)
3. ... *evaṃ soḷasavatthukaṃ ānāpānassatikammaṭṭhānaṃ niddiṭṭhaṃ* (... एवं सोळसवत्थुकं आनापानस्सतिकम्मट्ठानं निद्दिट्ठं.... ।) (Visuddhi. विसुद्धि० – VIII. 145).
4. "*Ānāpānassati, bhikkhave, bhāvitā bahulīkatā mahapphalā hoti mahānisaṃsā. Ānāpānassati, bhikkhave, bhāvitā bahulīkatā cattāro satipaṭṭhāne paripūrenti. Cattāro satipaṭṭhānā bhāvitā bahulīkatā satta bojjhaṅge paripūrenti. Satta bojjhaṅgā bhāvitā bahulīkatā vijjāvimuttiṃ paripūrenti.*" ("आनापानस्सति, भिक्खवे, भाविता बहुलीकता महप्फला होति महानिसंसा। आनापानस्सति, भिक्खवे, भाविता बहुलीकता चत्तारो सतिपट्ठाने परिपूरेन्ति। चत्तारो सतिपट्ठाना भाविता बहुलीकता सत्त बोज्झङ्गे परिपूरेन्ति। सत्त बोज्झङ्गा भाविता बहुलीकता विज्जाविमुत्तिं परिपूरेन्ति।") (Majjhima, Upari-paṇṇāsakaṃ) मज्झिम० । उपरिपण्णासकं। 18.2.5)

provision has, however, been kept for working on any other subject of meditation suiting one's temperament.

The Buddha did not favour verbalization of any sort as advocated by Patanjali.[1]

• Development of 'Samādhis' –

Patanjali categorises the states of samādhi according to the nature of their accompanying awareness. He distinguishes between two classes of samādhi, the first covering all those yogic states which are connected with intuitive knowledge (*prajñā*) (प्रज्ञा) and the other devoid of any objective substratum and also transcending intuitive knowledge (*prajñā*) (प्रज्ञा).

The first category of samādhi is called *samprajñāta* (सम्प्रज्ञात) (i.e., with intuitive knowledge)[2] and has the following classifications :

1. *Vitarkānugata* (वितर्कानुगत) (i.e., accompanied by initial application of the mind to the object);
2. *Vicārānugata* (विचारानुगत) (i.e., accompanied by sustained attention to the object);
3. *Ānandānugata* (आनन्दानुगत) (i.e., accompanied by joy or bliss); and
4. *Asmitānugata* (अस्मितानुगत) (i.e., accompanied by a sense-of-personality).

The second category has two phases, out of which the first one has not been given any name and is just called 'the other one' (*anyaḥ*) (अन्य:)[3] which seems to imply a samādhi beyond

---

1. Y.S. (I.28)
2. *Vitarkavicārānandāsmitārūpānugamāt samprajñātaḥ.* (वितर्कविचारानन्दास्मितारूपानुगमात्सम्प्रज्ञात: ॥) (Y.S. I.17)
3. *Virāmapratyayābhyāsapūrvaḥ saṃskāraśeṣo' nyaḥ.* (विरामप्रत्ययाभ्यासपूर्व: संस्कारशेषोऽन्य: ॥) (Y.S. I.18)

the stage of *samprajñāta* (सम्प्रज्ञात) (that is, the one with intuitive knowledge).[1] The samādhi of the second phase has been named *dharmamegha* (धर्ममेघ),[2] which represents the final stage before liberation.

In his quest for liberation, the aspirant has to attain the following stages :

(a) *Samāpatti-s* (समापत्ति) with concentration on thought-conception or rolling in thoughts (*savitarkā, savicārā*) (सवितर्का, सविचारा);

(b) *Samāpatti-s* (समापत्ति) without concentration on thought-conception or rolling in thoughts (*nirvitarkā, nirvicārā*) (निर्वितर्का, निर्विचारा), the latter having the following sub-stages :

(i) Samādhi accompanied by joy or bliss (*ānanda*) (आनन्द); and

(ii) Samādhi accompanied by sense-of-personality (*asmitā*) (अस्मिता);

(c) the functioning of intuitive knowledge (*prajñā*) (प्रज्ञा); and

(d) suppression of even *prajñā* (प्रज्ञा) (resulting in total cessation of mental processes).

---

1. This has the residue of a few subliminal impressions (*saṃskāra-s*) (संस्कार). In this respect it is comparable to the 'samādhi' producing the stage of a *sotāpanna*) (सोतापन्न) (stream-enterer) in the Buddha's teaching. In this also there is the residue of only a few subliminal impressions (सङ्खार) of higher planes of consciousness which remain to be eliminated for attaining the state of Full Enlightenment (Arhanthood).
2. *Prasaṅkhyāne' pyakusīdasya sarvathā vivekakhyāter - dharmameghaḥ samādhiḥ.* (प्रसंख्यानेऽप्यकुसीदस्य सर्वथा विवेकख्यातेर्धर्ममेघः समाधिः ॥) (Y.S. IV.29).

The samādhi of the last stage has been called 'seedless' (*nirbīja*) (निर्बीज)[1] while the rest of them have been named 'with seed' (*sabīja*) (सबीज).[2] The term '*seed*' (बीज) implies potentiality for formation of subliminal impressions (*saṃskāra-s*) (संस्कार). No such impression can be formed in the stage of the seedless (*nirbīja*) (निर्बीज) samādhi.

In terms of the Buddha's teaching, the samādhi 'with seed' (*sabīja*) (सबीज) would be one in which there are still latent-biases (*anusaya-kilesa-s*) (अनुसय-किलेस) in the mind. When all such latent-biases are cleared out, the samādhi would be 'seedless' (*nirbīja*) (निर्बीज), because no new subliminal impressions can be formed in this state of the mind.

According to his teaching, however, there are ten types of broad classifications of samādhi,[3] none of which is called 'with seed' (*sabīja*) (सबीज) or 'seedless' (*nirbīja*) (निर्बीज). Ideologically, however, these can be compared to *lokiya* (लोकिय) (mundane) and *lokuttara* (लोकुत्तर) (super-mundane) samādhis, respectively. The lokuttara samādhi (लोकुत्तर समाधि) has Nibbāna for its object. Any other samādhi, howsoever sublime, is merely *lokiya* (लोकिय) (mundane) in nature.

In this system, the following eight successive states (*samāpatti-s*) (समापत्ति) are induced by ecstatic meditation : -

1. Ist Absorption
2. IInd Absorption
3. IIIrd Absorption
4. IVth Absorption
5. Vth Absorption (in the sphere of Boundless Space)

---

1. *Tasyāpi nirodhe sarvanirodhānnirbījaḥ samādhiḥ* (तस्यापि निरोधे सर्वनिरोधान्निर्बीजः समाधिः ॥) (Y.S. I.51)
2. *Tā eva sabījaḥ samādhiḥ.* (ता एव सबीजः समाधिः ॥) (Y.S.I.46)
3. *Paṭisambhidā.* पटिसम्भिदा० (1.1.3.106)

6. VIth Absorption (in the sphere of Boundless Consciousness)
7. VIIth Absorption (in the sphere of Boundless Nothingness)
8. VIIIth Absorption (in the sphere of Neither-Perception-nor- Non-perception).[1]

From these one passes on to the stage of samādhi called *saññā-vedayita-nirodha* (सञ्ञा-वेदयित-निरोध) (i.e., extinction of perception and sensations). In this the aspirant realises supreme happiness and peace *(paramaṃ sukhaṃ, santi varapadaṃ)* (परमं सुखं, सन्ति वरपदं). The Buddha proclaimed that this samādhi was the highest one in which all the defiling impulses (*āsava-s*) (आसव) stand dwindled (*parikkhīṇā*) (परिक्खीणा).[2] This is the only samādhi which is super-mundane (*lokuttara*) (लोकुत्तर), all the rest being mundane (*lokiya*) (लोकिय).[3]

---

1. In the Pali Canon these are called – *paṭhama jhāna, dutiya jhāna, tatiya jhāna, catuttha jhāna, ākāsānañcāyatana samādhi, viññāṇañcāyatana samādhi, ākiñcaññāyatana samādhi* and *nevasaññānāsaññāyatana samādhi* (पठम झान, दुतिय झान, ततिय झान, चतुत्थ झान, आकासानञ्चायतन समाधि, विञ्ञाणञ्चायतन समाधि, आकिञ्चञ्ञायतन समाधि and नेवसञ्ञानासञ्ञायतन समाधि).
2. *Bhikkhu sabbaso nevasaññānāsaññāyatanaṃ samatikkamma saññāvedayitanirodhaṃ upasampajja viharati. Paññāya cassa disvā āsavā parikkhīṇā honti.* (भिक्खु सब्बसो नेवसञ्ञानासञ्ञायतनं समतिक्कम्म सञ्ञावेदयितनिरोधं उपसम्पज्ज विहरति। पञ्ञाय चस्स दिस्वा आसवा परिक्खीणा होन्ति।) (Majjhima, Mūla-paṇṇāsakaṃ मज्झिम० । मूलपण्णासकं।25.2.11)
3. The Buddha has stated that in the super-mundane state he remained conscious within but neither saw nor heard the streaming and splashing of the rain-god, flashing of lightning and crashing of thunder!

   Cf. Acchariyaṃ vata bho, abbhutaṃ vata bho, santena vata bho pabbajitā vihārena viharanti, yatra hi nāma saññī samāno jāgaro deve vassante gaḷagaḷāyante vijjullatāsu niccharantīsu asaniyā phaḷantiyā neva dakkhati na pana saddaṃ sossati. (अच्छरियं वत भो, अब्भुतं वत भो,

According to the Buddha, it was possible to attain *nirodhasamāpatti* (निरोधसमापत्ति) by undergoing the first four Absorptions only. With the help of intuitive knowledge (*paññā*) (पञ्ञा), it becomes possible to experience the truth of impermanence (that is, the arising and passing away of mind-matter phenomena) vividly till the IIIrd Absorption is attained. At its culminating stage one becomes firmly established in *sati* (सति) and *sampajañña* (सम्पजञ्ञ) (i.e., the faculties of mindfulness and constant thorough realisation of impermanence). While still working with these faculties in the path of the IVth Absorption, one attains 'extinction' (*nirodha*) (निरोध) at its culminating stage.

Meditative experience —

As already mentioned, the Yoga-Sutras describe two types of samādhis : one with intuitive knowledge (called *samprajñāta* सम्प्रज्ञात) and the other *anyaḥ* (अन्य:) transcending this one.[1]

Construed according to the Pali language, the term *samprajñāta* (सम्प्रज्ञात) would mean 'with sampajaññā.' *Sampajañña* (सम्पजञ्ञ) (Skt. सम्प्रज्ञान) is a technical term generally translated as 'clear comprehension', but this does not convey its real significance. Its real meaning is 'thorough realisation of impermanence in all bodily and mental activities at all times.'[2] The Buddha stressed quite frequently that a

सन्तेन वत भो पब्बजिता विहारेन विहरन्ति, यत्र हि नाम सञ्ञी समानो जागरो देवे वस्सन्ते गळगळायन्ते विज्जुल्लतासु निच्छरन्तीसु असनिया फलन्तिया नेव दक्खति न पन सद्दं सोस्सति! (Dīgha. Mahāvaggo. दीघ० । महावग्गो । 3.21.66)

1. Y.S. (1.17-18)
2. This means one should develop constant thorough realisation while walking, standing, sitting, sleeping, waking, chewing, eating, drinking, savouring, wearing clothes, attending to calls of nature and what not. (*Dīgha. Mahāvaggo* दीघ० । महावग्गो 9.2.5)
   If the continuous *sampajañña* (सम्पजञ्ञ) consists only of the thorough realisation of the processes involved in walking, standing, etc. then it is merely *sati* (सति) (*i.e.*, awareness, mindfulness). If the

meditator should not lose the thorough realisation of impermanence even for a moment.[1] For a meditator who followed his advice on the proper practice of Vipassanā, i.e., remaining *sampajāno* (सम्पजानो) without any interruption, he extended the assurance that the meditator will attain either the highest stage (Arahanthood) or the penultimate stage (Anāgāmitā).[2]

Thus, according to the Buddha's teaching, it is the constant thorough realisation of impermanence (*aniccatā*) (Skt. अनित्यता) of the mind-matter phenomena which paves the way for Full Enlightenment. While doing so, a meditator knows sensations arising in him, knows their persisting, and knows their vanishing; he knows initial applications (of the mind to objects) arising in him, knows their persisting, and knows their vanishing; he knows perceptions arising in him, knows their persisting, and knows their vanishing.[3]

As already mentioned at page 56, in the Yoga-Sutras one comes across use of the words *abhibhava-prādurbhāvau*

---

continuous *sampajañña* (सम्पजञ्ञ) includes observation of the characteristic of arising and passing away (*udayabbaya*) (उदयब्बय) of sensations (*vedanā*) (वेदना) while these activities are being performed, then it is real *sampajañña* (सम्पजञ्ञ), because then *paññā* (पञ्ञा) (wisdom) is at work. It was this type of *sampajañña* (सम्पजञ्ञ) which the Buddha wanted people to practise.

1. *Yato ca bhikkhu ātāpī, sampajaññaṃ na riñcati.* (यतो च भिक्खु आतापी, सम्पजञ्ञं न रिञ्चति।) (*Saṃyutta.* संयुत्त॰ - 36.12.12).
2. *Dīgha. Mahāvaggo* दीघ॰ । महावग्गो। - 9.6.33
3. *Idha, bhikkhave, bhikkhuno viditā vedanā uppajjanti, viditā upaṭṭhahanti, viditā abbhatthaṃ gacchanti. Viditā vitakkā uppajjanti, viditā upaṭṭhahanti, viditā abbhatthaṃ gacchanti. Viditā saññā uppajjanti, viditā upaṭṭhahanti, viditā abbhatthaṃ gacchanti.* (इध, भिक्खवे, भिक्खुनो विदिता वेदना उप्पज्जन्ति, विदिता उपट्ठहन्ति, विदिता अब्भत्थं गच्छन्ति। विदिता वितक्का उप्पज्जन्ति, विदिता उपट्ठहन्ति, विदिता अब्भत्थं

('अभिभव - प्रादुर्भावौ')[1] (dissolution and evolution), *kṣayodayau* ('क्षयोदयौ')[2] (fall and rise) and *śāntoditau* ('शान्तोदितौ')[3] (disappearance and appearance) which seem to signify the same thing as 'arising and passing away' in the Buddha's expositions. But this usage has nowhere been linked with the sensations (*vedanā*) (वेदना) where all mental states have their confluence.[4] The word *vedana* (वेदन) occurs but once in the Yoga-Sutras and that too in an entirely different context.[5] This only goes to show that the author of the Yoga-Sutras has missed this most important link of observing impermanence of the mind-matter phenomena at the level of sensations which is a serious lacuna in the path of Full Liberation.

The Yoga-Sutras, no doubt, mention the arising of the truth-bearing intuitive knowledge (*prajñā*) (प्रज्ञा) at the stage of the *nirvicāra samādhi* (निर्विचार समाधि)[6] (that is, without sustained attention to the object), but this knowledge does not seem to go so deep as to reveal the phenomenon of arising and passing away at the level of the sensations as mentioned above. The most plausible reason for this could be that the author of this work did not experience the truth of impermanence

---

गच्छन्ति। विदिता सञ्ञा उप्पज्जन्ति, विदिता उपट्ठहन्ति, विदिता अब्भत्थं गच्छन्ति।) (*Saṃyutta.* संयुत्त॰ - 47.35.38)

1. *Vyutthānanirodhasaṃskārayorabhibhavaprādurbhāvau nirodhakṣanacittānvayo nirodhapariṇāmaḥ.* (व्युत्थाननिरोधसंस्कारयोरभिभवप्रादुर्भावौ निरोधक्षणचित्तान्वयो निरोधपरिणामः॥) (Y.S. III.9)
2. *Sarvārthataikāgratayoḥ kṣayodayau cittassa samādhipariṇāmaḥ.* (सर्वार्थतैकाग्रतयोः क्षयोदयौ चित्तस्य समाधिपरिणामः॥) (Y.S. III. 11)
3. *Tataḥ punaḥ śāntoditau tulyapratyayau cittasyaikāgratā-pariṇāmaḥ.* (ततः पुनः शान्तोदितौ तुल्यप्रत्ययौ चित्तस्यैकाग्रतापरिणामः॥) (Y.S. III.12)
4. *Vedanā samosaraṇā sabbe dhammā* (वेदना समोसरणा सब्बे धम्मा।) (Aṅguttara. अङ्गुत्तर॰ - 10.6.8)
5. *Tataḥ prātibhaśrāvaṇavedanādarśāsvādavārtā jāyante.* (ततः प्रातिभश्रावणवेदनादर्शास्वादवार्ता जायन्ते॥) (Y.S. III.36)
6. Y.S. (I. 47-48)

himself and, bereft of such an experience, he came to hold some different notion of what "Truth" implies.

The Buddha's teaching provides for two branches of mental development (*bhāvanā*) (भावना), viz. 'Tranquillity' (*samatha*) (समथ) and 'Insight' (*vipassanā*) (विपस्सना), which are identical with 'concentration' (*samādhi*) (समाधि) and 'wisdom' (*paññā*) (पञ्ञा), respectively. 'Tranquillity', which can also be expressed as *passaddhi* पस्सद्धि) (Skt. *praśrabdhi* प्रश्रब्धि), is an unperturbed, peaceful and lucid state of mind attained by strong mental concentration. 'Insight' is the penetrative understanding, by direct meditative experience, of impermanence, unsatisfactoriness and impersonality, of all mental and material phenomena of existence. 'Insight' leads to entrance into the super-mundane states of Purity and to final liberation.[1]

There can be no 'insight' till one starts experiencing the truth of impermanence at the level of the bodily sensations.

---

1. 'Insight' develops as the mind becomes purer and purer. The path of purification lies through intuitive experience of impermanence, un-satisfactoriness and impersonality of all formations. Cf. -
Sabbe saṅkhārā aniccā ti, yadā paññāya passati,
atha nibbindati dukkhe, esa maggo visuddhiyā.
Sabbe saṅkhārā dukkhā ti, yadā paññāya passati,
atha nibbindati dukkhe, esa maggo visuddhiyā.
Sabbe dhammā anattā ti, yadā paññāya passati,
atha nibbindati dukkhe, esa maggo visuddhiyā.
(सब्बे सङ्खारा अनिच्चा ति, यदा पञ्ञाय पस्सति।
अथ निब्बिन्दति दुक्खे, एस मग्गो विसुद्धिया॥
सब्बे सङ्खारा दुक्खा ति, यदा पञ्ञाय पस्सति।
अथ निब्बिन्दति दुक्खे, एस मग्गो विसुद्धिया॥
सब्बे धम्मा अनत्ता ति, यदा पञ्ञाय पस्सति।
अथ निब्बिन्दति दुक्खे, एस मग्गो विसुद्धिया॥) (*Theragāthā* थेरगाथा-15.1.676-678)

Bodily sensations provide the nexus where the entire mind and body are tangibly revealed as an impermanent phenomenon leading to liberation. In its absence, one continues to remain in the realm of 'tranquillity'. 'Tranquillity' leads to development of the mind and abandonment of lust. 'Insight' leads to the development of wisdom and abandonment of ignorance.[1]

The aspirants, working according to the tenets of the Yoga-Sutras, do not penetrate their mind up to the level of the sensations which process gets into full stride from the IIIrd Absorption (*tatiyajjhāna*) (ततियज्झान) onwards in the case of the Buddha's teaching. As a result of this, they cannot reach the culmination stage of the IIIrd Absorption and, remaining in the realm of 'Tranquillity', can, at the most, benefit by abandoning their lust. It is inconceivable that they can come out of Ignorance (*avijjā*) (अविज्जा) in the real sense of the term in spite of their claim in this regard, unless they experience the (impermanent nature of) sensations on a non-stop basis (Pali *sampajañña* सम्पजञ्ञ, Skt. *Samprajñāna* सम्प्रज्ञान). (For a detailed explanation of this term, please see the ANNEXURE).

• Need for a step beyond Yoga —

The desideratum of Yoga is to experience the cessation of mental fluctuations (*cittavṛttinirodhaḥ*) (चित्तवृत्तिनिरोध:). The

---

1. *Samatho, bhikkhave, bhāvito kamatthamanubhoti? Cittaṃ bhāvīyati. Cittaṃ bhāvitaṃ kamatthamanubhoti? Yo rāgo so pahīyati. Vipassanā, bhikkhave, bhāvitā kamatthamanubhoti ? Paññā bhāvīyati. Paññā bhāvitā kamatthamanubhoti? Yā avijjā sā pahīyati.* (समथो, भिक्खवे, भावितो कमत्थमनुभोति? चित्तं भावीयति। चित्तं भावितं कमत्थमनुभोति? यो रागो सो पहीयति। विपस्सना, भिक्खवे, भाविता कमत्थमनुभोति? पञ्ञा भावीयति। पञ्ञा भाविता कमत्थमनुभोति? या अविज्जा सा पहीयति।) (*Aṅguttara* अङ्गुत्तर० - 2.3.11)

Buddha's teaching makes one experience the cessation of the mind itself (*cittanirodha*) (चित्तनिरोध). Thus, there is need for taking a step beyond Yoga.[1]

---

1. The views expressed by Ernst E. Wood on this subject deserve attention :
"Orthodox Yoga quietens the ego but does not kill its dominance; to achieve this last indispensable task it is needful to go a step beyond Yoga. The ego itself is so cunning, its wiles are so clever and tricky that the average yogi is easily deceived into believing it to be subdued when, in fact, it is merely biding its time. Gautam the Buddha had to take this step and tread this ultimate path."
(Practical Yoga — Ancient and Modern)

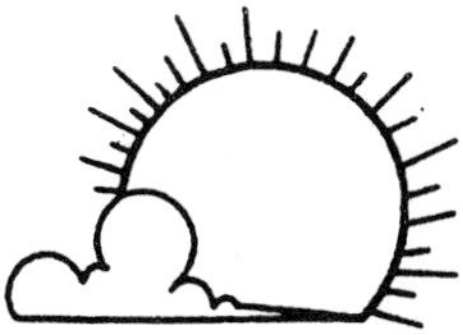

SECTION - V

THE TASTE OF THE PUDDING IS IN THE EATING

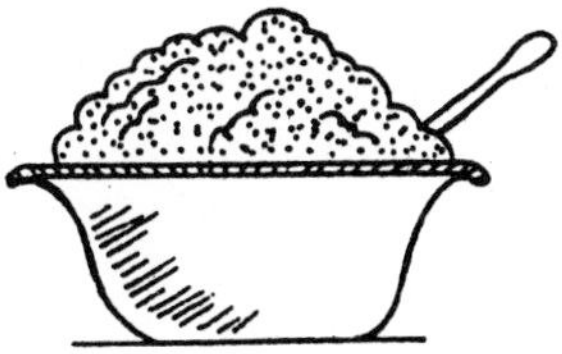

According to the Yoga-Sutras, with the attainment of the *dharmamegha* (धर्ममेघ) samādhi, all afflictions (*kleśa-s*) (क्लेश) and deeds (*karma-s*) (कर्म) come to an end[1] and the primary energies (*guṇa-s*) (गुण) revert to the transcendent core of Nature. This constitutes the state of Isolation (*kaivalya*) (कैवल्य) and the Puruṣa begins to shine in full splendour.[2] The yogi now stands fully liberated from his cycles of birth and death.

The Buddha also taught the technique of *vipassanā* (विपस्सना) meditation for eradicating all the mental impurities so as to make the mind ultra-pure. The practical steps of this technique are contained in the Fourfold Satipaṭṭhāna[3] (*cattāro satipaṭṭhānā*) (चत्तारो सतिपट्ठाना). These are : constant observation of the body (*kāyānupassanā*) (कायानुपस्सना), constant observation of sensations (*vedanānupassanā*) (वेदनानुपस्सना), constant observation of mind (*cittānupassanā*) (चित्तानुपस्सना) and constant observation of the contents of the mind (*dhammānupassanā*) (धम्मानुपस्सना). The Buddha proclaimed this as the only path for the purification of beings, for going beyond sorrow and lamentation, for the extinguishing of

1. *Tataḥ kleśakarmanivṛttiḥ* (ततः क्लेशकर्मनिवृत्तिः ॥) (Y.S. IV.30)
2. *Puruśārthaśūnyānāṃ guṇānāṃ pratiprasavaḥ kaivalyaṃ svarūpapratiṣṭhā vā citiśaktiriti* (पुरुषार्थशून्यानां गुणानां प्रतिप्रसवः कैवल्यं स्वरूपप्रतिष्ठा वा चितिशक्तिरिति ॥) (Y.S. IV.34)
3. '*Satipaṭṭhāna*' means 'establishing of awareness or mindfulness'.

suffering and grief, for walking on the path of truth, for the realisation of Nibbāna —[1] the *summum bonum* of all existence.

A question now arises whether the person who followed this or that teaching could achieve the goal laid down therein. Obviously, the taste of the pudding would lie in the eating. While we have not come across any instance where the practitioner has come forward to proclaim that he or she had attained the state of isolation (*kaivalya*) (कैवल्य) as described in the Yoga-Sutras, there are any number of persons who, following the teaching of the Buddha, were able to attain the state of non-return to the worldly existence and proclaimed this fact as such. Here are a few instances :

(a) Uttarapāla, the Elder proclaims all his desires have dissipated, all types of existences destroyed, the thread of successive lives thrown to the winds, with the result that there is now no new birth in store for him.[2]

(b) Nhātaka-muni, the Elder states all the five aggregates have been known comprehensively, with their roots cut asunder, the end of sufferings has been sighted and now there is no new birth in store for him.[3]

---

1. *'Ekāyano ayaṃ, bhikkhave, maggo sattānaṃ visuddhiyā, sokaparidevānaṃ samatikkamāya dukkhadomanassānaṃ atthaṅgamāya, ñāyassa adhigamāya, nibbānassa sacchikiriyāya — yadidaṃ cattāro satipaṭṭhānā.'*
   ('एकायनो अयं, भिक्खवे, मग्गो सत्तानं विसुद्धिया, सोकपरिदेवानं समतिक्कमाय, दुक्खदोमनस्सानं अत्थङ्गमाय, ञायस्स अधिगमाय, निब्बानस्स सच्छिकिरियाय - यदिदं चत्तारो सतिपट्ठाना।') (*Dīgha. Mahāvaggo* दीघ० । महावग्गो । 9.1.2)
2. *Sabbe kāmā pahīnā me, bhavā sabbe padālitā; vikkhīṇo jātisaṃsāro, natthi dāni punabbhavo.*
   (सब्बे कामा पहीना मे, भवा सब्बे पदालिता।
   विक्खीणो जातिसंसारो, नत्थि दानि पुनब्भवो॥) (*Theragāthā.* थेरगाथा - 3.12.254)
3. *Pañcakkhandhā pariññātā, tiṭṭhanti chinnamūlakā; dukkhakkhayo anuppatto, natthi dāni punabbhavo.*
   (पञ्चक्खन्धा परिञ्ञाता, तिट्ठन्ति छिन्नमूलका।
   दुक्खक्खयो अनुप्पत्तो, नत्थि दानि पुनब्भवो॥) (*Theragāthā.* थेरगाथा

(c) Madhudāyaka, the Elder asserts he has transgressed all the worldly existences — whether middling, superior or inferior — this day all his defiling impulses stand dwindled and now there is no new birth in store for him.[1]

(d) Hemakattha, the Elder says this is his last, last worldly existence, all his defiling impulses have come to an end and now there is no new life in store for him.[2]

(e) Mañcadāyaka, the Elder declares all his sins stand roasted, all worldly existences up-rooted, all the defiling impulses destroyed and now there is no new birth in store for him.[3]

(f) Ekasaniya, the Elder affirms the three-fold fires within him stand extinguished, all the corporeal existences stand vanquished, this is his last mundane existence in the Dispensation of the Perfectly Enlightened One.[4]

6.11.440)

1. *Majjhe mahante hīne ca, bhave sabbe atikkamiṃ; ajja me āsavā khīṇā, natthi dāni punabbavo..*
(मज्झे महन्ते हीने च, भवे सब्बे अतिक्कमिं।
अज्ज मे आसवा खीणा, नत्थि दानि पुनब्भवो॥) (*Therāpadāna.* थेरापदान - 40.4.348)

2. *Idaṃ pacchimakaṃ mayhaṃ, carimo vattate bhavo; sabbāsavā parikkhīṇā, natthi dāni punabbhavo.*
(इदं पच्छिमकं मय्हं, चरिमो वत्तते भवो॥
सब्बासवा परिक्खीणा, नत्थि दानि पुनब्भवो॥) (*Therāpadāna.* थेरापदान - 41.7.220)

3. *Kilesā jhāpitā mayhaṃ, bhavā sabbe samūhatā; sabbāsavā parikkhīṇā, natthi dāni punabbhavo.*
(किलेसा झापिता मय्हं, भवा सब्बे समूहता।
सब्बासवा परिक्खीणा, नत्थि दानि पुनब्भवो॥) (*Therāpadāna.* थेरापदान - 13.2.16)

4. *Tividhaggī nibbutā mayhaṃ, bhavā sabbe samūhatā; dhāremi antimaṃ dehaṃ, sammāsambuddhasāsane.*
(तिविधग्गी निब्बुता मय्हं, भवा सब्बे समूहता।
धारेमि अन्तिमं देहं, सम्मासम्बुद्धसासने॥) (*Therāpadāna* थेरापदान - 12.4.37)

(g) Bhaddāli, the Elder acclaims this is his very last worldly existence and that he is moving about without any defiling impulses like an elephant having shattered all fetters ![1]

(h) Kāḷudāyī, the Elder comes out with a proclamation that all his cravings, aversions, delusions, pride and envy stand vanquished and, having known all his defiling impulses down to the roots, he now moves about without any such impulse.[2]

(i) Ugga, the Elder avers whatever Kamma — small or great — had been performed by him, all that has come to an end. There is now no new birth in store for him.[3]

(J) Eka-piṇḍa-pāta-dāyikā, the she-Elder is filled with a paean of joy while acclaiming that now she is free from all fetters, her limiting adjuncts have all disappeared, all her defiling impulses have exhausted and now there is no new birth in store for her.[4]

(k) Udaka-dāyikā, the she-Elder says exultingly today she is having an intrinsically pure mind, all the sinful factors having been cast off by the mind, she has liquidated all her defiling impulses and now there is no

---

1. *Idaṃ pacchimakaṃ mayhaṃ, carimo vattate bhavo; nāgo va bandhanaṃ chetvā, viharāmi anāsavo.*
(इदं पच्छिमकं मय्हं, चरिमो वत्तते भवो।
नागो व बन्धनं छेत्वा, विहरामि अनासवो॥) (*Therāpadāna* थेरापदान - 42.1.28)
2. *Rāgo doso ca moho ca, māno makkho ca dhaṃsito; sabbāsave pariññāya, viharāmi anāsavo.*
(रागो दोसो च मोहो च, मानो मक्खो च धंसितो।
सब्बासवे परिञ्ञाय, विहरामि अनासवो॥) (*Therāpadāna* थेरापदान - 4.4.61)
3. *Yaṃ mayā pakataṃ kammaṃ, appaṃ vā yadi vā bahuṃ; sabbametaṃ parikkhīṇaṃ, natthi dāni punabbhavo.*
(यं मया पकतं कम्मं, अप्पं वा यदि वा बहुं।
सब्बमेतं परिक्खीणं, नत्थि दानि पुनब्भवो॥) (*Theragāthā* थेरगाथा - 1.80.80)
4. *Sabbabandhanamuttāhaṃ, apetā me upādikā; sabbāsavaparikkhīṇā, natthi dāni punabbhavo.*
(सब्बबन्धनमुत्ताहं, अपेता मे उपादिका।
सब्बासवपरिक्खीणा, नत्थि दानि पुनब्भवो॥) (*Therī-apadāna* थेरीअपदान-1.6.55)

new life in store for her.[1]

Besides the above, there are a large number of other persons who have, in a similar vein, proclaimed about the highest achievement in the Dispensation of the Buddha. Paṭācārā, for example, compares the experience of her emancipation to the extinction of a burning flame.[2] Sumedhā speaks about her direct realization of the Six-fold Higher Knowledge.[3] Kisā-gotamī speaks about her direct experience of Nibbāna.[4] Khemā tells about her release from all sufferings.[5]

---

1. *Visuddhamanasā ajja, apetamanapāpikā; sabbāsavaparikkhīṇā, natthi dāni punabbhavo.* (विसुद्धमनसा अज्ज, अपेतमनपापिका। सब्बासवपरिक्खीणा, नत्थि दानि पुनब्भवो॥) (*Therī-apadāna* थेरीअपदान - 1.10.126)
2. *Padīpasseva nibbānaṃ, vimokkho ahu cetaso.* (पदीपस्सेव निब्बानं, विमोक्खो अहु चेतसो।) (*Therīgāthā.* थेरीगाथा - 5.10.116)
3. *Cha abhiññā sacchikatā, aggaphalaṃ sikkhamānāya.* (छ अभिञ्ञा सच्छिकता, अग्गफलं सिक्खमानाय।) (*Therīgāthā.* थेरीगाथा - 16.1.518)
4. *Nibbānaṃ sacchikataṃ, dhammādāsaṃ avekkhihaṃ.* (निब्बानं सच्छिकतं, धम्मादासं अवेक्खिहं।) (*Therīgāthā.* थेरीगाथा -10.1.222)
5. *Pamuttā sabbadukkhehi, satthusāsanakārikā.* (पमुत्ता सब्बदुक्खेहि, सत्थुसासनकारिका।) (*Therīgāthā.* थेरीगाथा - 6.3.144)

Sampajañña

There are several technical terms in Pali which are of significance both in the field of *pariyatti* (theory) and *paṭipatti* (practice). One such word is *sampajañña*. This term often occurs along with *sati* in the expressions *sati sampajaññaṃ*, or *sato ca sampajāno*, or *sato sampajāno*. As a result, it has been widely interpreted as an exhortation to be mindful and has been defined as being nearly synonymous with *sato*[1] (with awareness), merely indicating a greater intensity of awareness. However, the Abhidhamma texts suggest a different rendering of this word. In the *Dhammasaṅgaṇi*, *Vibhaṅga* and *Dhātukathā* we find the following definition of *sampajāno*:

> *"Sampajāno" ti tattha katamaṃ sampajaññaṃ ? Yā paññā pajānanā vicayo pavicayo dhammavicayo sallakkhaṇā upalakkhaṇā paccupalakkhaṇā paṇḍiccaṃ kosallaṃ nepuññaṃ vebhabyā cintā upaparikkhā bhūrīmedhā pariṇāyikā vipassanā sampajaññaṃ .... sammādiṭṭhi—idaṃ vuccati sampajaññaṃ.*[2]
>
> What is *sampajañña* ? That which is wisdom, understanding, investigation, deep investigation, truth investigation, discernment, discrimination, differentiation, erudition , proficiency, skill, analysis, consideration, close examination, breadth, sagacity, guidance, insight, thorough understanding of impermanence... right view — this is called *sampajañña.*

This plethora of nouns and metaphors clearly conveys that *sampajañña* is not awareness but wisdom. This definition is confirmed by the etymology of the word, formed by the addition of the prefix *saṃ*[3] to *pajānanā*[4], "knowing with wisdom." Rather it refers to an intensified kind of understanding : knowing correctly with wisdom or knowing in totality with thorough understanding. The exhortation of the

Buddha is to develop not simply awareness but also wisdom. That is why the text states :

Sampajaññan ti paññā.[5]

Sampajañña is wisdom.

The commentaries explain more precisely what *sampajañña* consists of :

Sammā pakārehi aniccādīni jānātīti sampajaññaṃ.

One who knows in a right way impermanence (as well as suffering and egolessness), has wisdom, *sampajañña.*[6]

Samantato pakārehi pakataṃ va savisesaṃ jānātīti sampajāno.[7]

One who understands the totality clearly with wisdom from all angles (of whatever is happening moment to moment), or who knows distinctly (the ultimate), has *sampajañña.*

The Buddha always taught that wisdom (*paññā*) is knowing things from different angles in the correct way. He used these descriptions : *sammā pakārehi - jānanaṃ* (seeing from different perspectives, in totality); *samantato pakārehi jānanaṃ* (having a complete and correct picture, so that nothing is left unseen and unknown);

Sammā samantato samañca pajānanto sampajāno.[7]

One who knows in a right way in totality through one's wisdom is *sampajāno*.

In particular, as meditators we must see not only the superficial, external appearances of things, that is, the apparent (*saṃvuti sacca*), but also the ultimate (*paramattha sacca*) or subtle understanding of reality. The apparent truth about the world and ourselves is that we exist as individual separate entities, but the ultimate is that every moment everything, both the world as well as ourselves, is in constant flux. This fact of impermanence has to be realized on the basis of experience and not merely at the intellectual level. It is only when we experience this reality of arising and passing away that we emerge from suffering (*dukkha*) and egotism (*attā*). This is what *sampajañña* enables us to do.

Therefore, for a meditator, *sampajañña* is complete understanding. It is insight into all aspects of the human phenomenon, mental as well as physical. We must understand that whenever the mind encounters an object, it perceives and evaluates it in a distorted way through the coloured lens of past conditioning; it therefore reacts with ignorance, craving or aversion. This is the process that produces suffering, because wisdom is lacking.

Mind is reflected in the body and it is through its physical manifestation that we can clearly grasp its nature of arising and passing away. This is why we find in the *Mahāsatipaṭṭhāna-sutta* that the paragraph on *sampajañña* is contained in the section on the observation of body (*Kāyānupassanā*). To realize the fact of impermanence of our bodily activities, we must experience them at the level of sensations (*vedanā*) felt within the body. At a deep intuitive level these enable us to recognize our ephemeral nature.

Thus *sampajañña* is the realization of our own ephemeral nature at the deepest level. Far from being an equivalent of *sati*, it is the complement of *sati*.

The uniting of these two faculties is *satipaṭṭhāna*, the establishing of awareness, by means of which we can reach the goal of freedom from suffering.

Notes

1. See, for example, *Pali-English Dictionary*, ed. T.W. Rhys Davids, Pali Text Society, London, 1925, entries for *sampajañña* and *sampajāno*.
2. *Dhammasaṅgaṇi*, Nal. 83, PTS 68; Vibhanga, Nal. 239, PTS 194; *Puggalapaññatti*, Nal. 41, PTS 40.
3. See *A Dictionary of the Pali Language* ed. R.C. Childers, Kegan Paul Ltd., London, 1909, p. 423, under entry for *sam*.
4. *pa* + *jānana* = *pajānana* - know with wisdom.
5. *Abhidhamma aṭṭhakathā* II. 133 (Burmese Edition)
6. *Abhidhamma aṭṭhakathā* I, 192 (Burmese Edition); *Paṭisambhidāmagga aṭṭhakathā*, 343 (Burmese Edition).
7. *Dīgha-nikāya ṭīkā II*, 81 (Burmese Edition).

PATANJALI'S YOGA-SUTRAS

CHAPTER - I

1. Atha Yogānuśāsanam.
अथ योगानुशासनम् ।

2. Yogaścittavṛttinirodhaḥ.
योगश्चित्तवृत्तिनिरोधः ।

3. Tadā draṣṭuḥ svarūpe' vasthānam.
तदा द्रष्टुः स्वरूपेऽवस्थानम् ।

4. Vṛttisārūpyamitaratra.
वृत्तिसारूप्यमितरत्र ।

5. Vṛttayaḥ pañcatayyaḥ kliṣṭākliṣṭāḥ.
वृत्तयः पञ्चतय्यः क्लिष्टाक्लिष्टाः ।

6. Pramāṇaviparyayavikalpanidrāsmṛtayaḥ.
प्रमाणविपर्ययविकल्पनिद्रास्मृतयः ।

7. Pratyakṣānumānāgamāḥ pramāṇāni.
प्रत्यक्षानुमानागमाः प्रमाणानि ।

8. Viparyayo mithyājñānamatadrūpapratiṣṭham.
विपर्ययो मिथ्याज्ञानमतद्रूपप्रतिष्ठम् ।

9. Śabdajñānānupātī vastuśūnyo vikalpaḥ.
शब्दज्ञानानुपाती वस्तुशून्यो विकल्पः ।

10. Abhāvapratyayālambanā vṛttirnidrā.
अभावप्रत्ययालम्बना वृत्तिर्निद्रा ।

11. Anubhūtaviśayāsampramoṣaḥ smṛtiḥ.
अनुभूतविषयासंप्रमोषः स्मृतिः।

12. Abhyāsavairāgyābhyāṃ tannirodhaḥ.
अभ्यासवैराग्याभ्यां तन्निरोधः।

13. Tatra sthitau yatno' bhyāsaḥ.
तत्र स्थितौ यत्नोऽभ्यासः।

14. Sa tu dīrghakālanairantaryasatkārāsevito dṛḍhabhūmiḥ.
स तु दीर्घकालनैरन्तर्यसत्कारासेवितो दृढभूमिः।

15. Dṛṣṭānuśravikaviṣayavitṛṣṇasya vaśīkārasaṃjñā vairāgyam.
दृष्टानुश्रविकविषयवितृष्णस्य वशीकारसंज्ञा वैराग्यम्।

16. Tatparaṃ puruṣakhyāterguṇavaitṛṣṇyam.
तत्परं पुरुषख्यातेर्गुणवैतृष्ण्यम्।

17. Vitarkavicārānandāsmitārūpānugamāt saṃprajñātaḥ.
वितर्कविचारानन्दास्मितारूपानुगमात् संप्रज्ञातः।

18. Virāmapratyayābhyāsapūrvaḥ saṃskāraśeṣo'nyaḥ.
विरामप्रत्ययाभ्यासपूर्वः संस्कारशेषोऽन्यः।

19. Bhavapratyayo videhaprakṛtilayānām.
भवप्रत्ययो विदेहप्रकृतिलयानाम्।

20. Śraddhāvīryasmṛtisamādhiprajñāpūrvaka itareṣām.
श्रद्धावीर्यस्मृतिसमाधिप्रज्ञापूर्वक इतरेषाम्।

21. Tīvrasaṃvegānāmāsannaḥ
तीव्रसंवेगानामासन्नः।

22. Mṛdumadhyādhimātratvāttato' pi viśeṣaḥ.
मृदुमध्याधिमात्रत्वात्ततोऽपि विशेषः।

23. Īśvarapraṇidhānād vā.
ईश्वरप्रणिधानाद् वा।

24. Kleśakarmavipākāśayairaparāmṛṣṭaḥ puruṣaviśeṣa Īśvaraḥ.
क्लेशकर्मविपाकाशयैरपरामृष्टः पुरुषविशेष ईश्वरः।

25. Tatra niratiśayaṃ sarvajñabījam.
तत्र निरतिशयं सर्वज्ञबीजम्।

26. Sa eṣa pūrveṣāmapi guruḥ kālenānavacchedāt.
स एष पूर्वेषामपि गुरुः कालेनानवच्छेदात्।

27. Tasya vācakaḥ praṇavaḥ.
तस्य वाचकः प्रणवः।

28. Tajjapastadarthabhāvanam.
तज्जपस्तदर्थभावनम्।

29. Tataḥ pratyakcetanādhigamo' pyantarāyābhāvaśca.
ततः प्रत्यक्चेतनाधिगमोऽप्यन्तरायाभावश्च।

30. Vyādhistyānasaṃśayapramādālasyāviratibhrāntidarśanālabdhabhūmikatvānavasthitatvāni cittavikṣepāste' ntarāyāḥ.
व्याधिस्त्यानसंशयप्रमादालस्याविरतिभ्रान्तिदर्शनालब्ध-
भूमिकत्वानवस्थितत्वानि चित्तविक्षेपास्तेऽन्तरायाः।

31. Duḥkhadaurmanasyāṅgamejayatvaśvāsapraśvāsā vikṣepasahabhuvaḥ.
दुःखदौर्मनस्याङ्गमेजयत्वश्वासप्रश्वासा विक्षेपसहभुवः।

32. Tatpratiṣedhārthamekatattvābhyāsaḥ.
तत्प्रतिषेधार्थमेकतत्त्वाभ्यासः।

33. Maitrīkaruṇāmuditopekṣāṇāṃ sukhaduḥkhapuṇyāpuṇyaviśayāṇāṃ bhāvanātaścitta-prasādanam.
मैत्रीकरुणामुदितोपेक्षाणां सुखदुःखपुण्यापुण्यविषयाणां भावनातश्चित्तप्रसादनम्।

34. Pracchardanavidhāraṇābhyāṃ vā prāṇasya.
प्रच्छर्दनविधारणाभ्यां वा प्राणस्य।

35. Viṣayavatī vā pravṛttirutpannā manasaḥ sthitinibandhinī.
विषयवती वा प्रवृत्तिरुत्पन्ना मनसः स्थितिनिबन्धिनी।

36. Viśokā vā jyotiṣmatī.
विशोका वा ज्योतिष्मती।

37. Vītarāgaviṣayaṃ vā cittam.
वीतरागविषयं वा चित्तम्।

38. Svapnanidrājñānālambanaṃ vā.
स्वप्ननिद्राज्ञानालम्बनं वा।

39. Yathābhimatadhyānād vā.
यथाभिमतध्यानाद् वा।

40. Paramāṇuparamamahatvānto'sya vaśīkāraḥ.
परमाणुपरममहत्त्वान्तोऽस्य वशीकारः।

41. Kṣīṇavṛtterabhijātasyeva maṇergrahītṛgrahaṇagrāhyeṣu tatsthatadañjanatā samāpattiḥ.
क्षीणवृत्तेरभिजातस्येव मणेर्ग्रहीतृग्रहणग्राह्येषु तत्स्थतदञ्जनता समापत्तिः।

42. Tatra śabdārthajñānavikalpaiḥ saṅkīrṇā savitarkā samāpattiḥ.

तत्र शब्दार्थज्ञानविकल्पैः सङ्कीर्णा सवितर्का समापत्तिः।

43. Smṛtipariśuddhau svarūpaśūnyevārthamātra-nirbhāsā nirvitarkā.

स्मृतिपरिशुद्धौ स्वरूपशून्येवार्थमात्रनिर्भासा निर्वितर्का।

44. Etayaiva savicārā nirvicārā ca sūkṣmaviṣayā vyākhyātā.

एतयैव सविचारा निर्विचारा च सूक्ष्मविषया व्याख्याता।

45. Sūkṣmaviṣayatvaṃ cāliṅgaparyavasānam.

सूक्ष्मविषयत्वं चालिङ्गपर्यवसानम्।

46. Tā eva sabījaḥ samādhiḥ.

ता एव सबीजः समाधिः।

47. Nirvicāravaiśāradye' dhyātmaprasādaḥ.

निर्विचारवैशारद्येऽध्यात्मप्रसादः।

48. Ṛtambharā tatra prajñā.

ऋतम्भरा तत्र प्रज्ञा।

49. Ṣrutānumānaprajñābhyāmanyaviṣayā viśeṣārthatvāt.

श्रुतानुमानप्रज्ञाभ्यामन्यविषया विशेषार्थत्वात्।

50. Tajjaḥ saṃskāro' nyasaṃskārapratibandhī.

तज्जः संस्कारोऽन्यसंस्कारप्रतिबन्धी।

51. Tasyāpi nirodhe sarvanirodhānnirbījaḥ samādhiḥ.

तस्यापि निरोधे सर्वनिरोधान्निर्बीजः समाधिः।

CHAPTER - II

1. Tapaḥsvādhyāyeśvarapraṇidhānāni kriyāyogaḥ.
   तपःस्वाध्यायेश्वरप्रणिधानानि क्रियायोगः।

2. Samādhibhāvanārthaḥ kleśatanūkaraṇārthaśca.
   समाधिभावनार्थः क्लेशतनूकरणार्थश्च।

3. Avidyāsmitārāgadveṣābhiniveśāḥ kleśāḥ.
   अविद्यास्मितारागद्वेषाभिनिवेशाः क्लेशाः।

4. Avidyākṣetramuttareṣāṃ prasuptatanu-vicchinnodārāṇām.
   अविद्याक्षेत्रमुत्तरेषां प्रसुप्ततनुविच्छिन्नोदाराणाम्।

5. Anityāśuciduḥkhānātmasu nityaśucisukhātma-khyātiravidyā.
   अनित्याशुचिदुःखानात्मसु नित्यशुचिसुखात्मख्यातिरविद्या।

6. Dṛgdarśanaśaktyorekātmatevāsmitā.
   दृग्दर्शनशक्त्योरेकात्मतेवास्मिता।

7. Sukhānuśayī rāgaḥ.
   सुखानुशयी रागः।

8. Duḥkhānuśayī dveṣaḥ.
   दुःखानुशयी द्वेषः।

9. Svarasavāhī viduṣo'pi tathārūḍho' bhiniveśaḥ.
   स्वरसवाही विदुषोऽपि तथारूढोऽभिनिवेशः।

10. Te pratiprasavaheyāḥ sūkṣmāḥ.
    ते प्रतिप्रसवहेयाः सूक्ष्माः।

11. Dhyānaheyāstadvṛttayaḥ.
    ध्यानहेयास्तद्वृत्तयः।

12. Kleśamūlaḥ karmāśayo dṛṣṭādṛṣṭajanmavedanīyaḥ.
क्लेशमूलः कर्माशयो दृष्टादृष्टजन्मवेदनीयः।

13. Sati mūle tadvipāko jātyāyurbhogāḥ.
सति मूले तद्विपाको जात्यायुर्भोगाः।

14. Te hlādaparitāpaphalāḥ puṇyāpuṇyahetutvāt.
ते ह्लादपरितापफलाः पुण्यापुण्यहेतुत्वात्।

15. Pariṇāmatāpasaṃskāraduḥkhairguṇavṛttivirodhācca duḥkhameva sarvaṃ vivekinaḥ.
परिणामतापसंस्कारदुःखैर्गुणवृत्तिविरोधाच्च दुःखमेव सर्वं विवेकिनः।

16. Heyaṃ duḥkhamanāgatam.
हेयं दुःखमनागतम्।

17. Draṣṭṛdṛśyayoḥ saṃyogo heyahetuḥ.
द्रष्टृदृश्ययोः संयोगो हेयहेतुः।

18. Prakāśakriyāsthitiśīlaṃ bhūtendriyātmakaṃ bhogāpavargārthaṃ dṛśyam.
प्रकाशक्रियास्थितिशीलं भूतेन्द्रियात्मकं भोगापवर्गार्थं दृश्यम्।

19. Viśeṣāviśeṣaliṅgamātrāliṅgāni guṇaparvāṇi.
विशेषाविशेषलिङ्गमात्रालिङ्गानि गुणपर्वाणि।

20. Draṣṭā dṛśimātraḥ śuddho'pi pratyayānupaśyaḥ.
द्रष्टा दृशिमात्रः शुद्धोऽपि प्रत्ययानुपश्यः।

21. Tadartha eva dṛśyasyātmā.
तदर्थ एव दृश्यस्यात्मा।

22. Kṛtārthaṃ prati naṣṭamapyanaṣṭaṃ tadanya-sādhāraṇatvāt.

कृतार्थं प्रति नष्टमप्यनष्टं तदन्यसाधारणत्वात्।

23. Svasvāmiśaktyoḥ svarūpopalabdhihetuḥ saṃyogaḥ.

स्वस्वामिशक्त्योः स्वरूपोपलब्धिहेतुः संयोगः।

24. Tasya heturavidyā.

तस्य हेतुरविद्या।

25. Tadabhāvāt saṃyogābhāvo hānaṃ tad dṛśeḥ kaivalyam.

तदभावात्संयोगाभावो हानं तद्दृशेः कैवल्यम्।

26. Vivekakhyātiraviplavā hānopāyaḥ.

विवेकख्यातिरविप्लवा हानोपायः ।

27. Tasya saptadhā prāntabhūmiḥ prajñā.

तस्य सप्तधा प्रान्तभूमिः प्रज्ञा।

28. Yogāṅgānuṣṭhānādaśuddhikṣaye jñānadīptirāvivekakhyāteḥ.

योगाङ्गानुष्ठानादशुद्धिक्षये ज्ञानदीप्तिराविवेकख्यातेः।

29. Yamaniyamāsanaprāṇāyāmapratyāhāradhāraṇādhy-ānasamādhayo' ṣṭāvaṅgāni.

यमनियमासनप्राणायामप्रत्याहारधारणाध्यानसमाधयोऽ
ष्टावङ्गानि।

30. Tatrāhiṃsāsatyāsteyabrahmacaryāparigrahā yamāḥ.

तत्राहिंसासत्यास्तेयब्रह्मचर्यापरिग्रहा यमाः।

31. Jātideśakālasamayānavacchinnāḥ sārvabhaumā mahāvratam.

जातिदेशकालसमयानवच्छिन्नाः सार्वभौमा महाव्रतम्।

32. Śaucasantoṣatapaḥsvādhyāyeśvarapraṇidhānāni niyamāḥ.

शौचसन्तोषतपःस्वाध्यायेश्वरप्रणिधानानि नियमाः।

33. Vitarkabādhane pratipakṣabhāvanam.

वितर्कबाधने प्रतिपक्षभावनम्।

34. Vitarkā hiṃsādayaḥ kṛtakāritānumoditā lobhakrodhamohapūrvakā mṛdumadhyādhimātrā duḥkhājñānānantaphalā iti pratipakṣabhāvanam.

वितर्का हिंसादयः कृतकारितानुमोदिता लोभक्रोधमोहपूर्वका मृदुमध्याधिमात्रा दुःखाज्ञानानन्तफला इति प्रतिपक्षभावनम्।

35. Ahiṃsāpratiṣṭhāyāṃ tatsannidhau vairatyāgaḥ.

अहिंसाप्रतिष्ठायां तत्सन्निधौ वैरत्यागः।

36. Satyapratiṣṭhāyāṃ kriyāphalāśrayatvam.

सत्यप्रतिष्ठायां क्रियाफलाश्रयत्वम्।

37. Asteyapratiṣṭhāyāṃ sarvaratnopasthānam.

अस्तेयप्रतिष्ठायां सर्वरत्नोपस्थानम्।

38. Brahmacaryapratiṣṭhāyāṃ vīryalābhaḥ.

ब्रह्मचर्यप्रतिष्ठायां वीर्यलाभः।

39. Aparigrahasthairye janmakathantā saṃbodhaḥ.

अपरिग्रहस्थैर्ये जन्मकथंता संबोधः॥

40. Śaucātsvāṅgajugupsā parairasaṃsargaḥ.

शौचात्स्वाङ्गजुगुप्सा परैरसंसर्गः।

41. Sattvaśuddhau saumanasyaikāgryendriyajayātmadarśanayogyatvāni ca.

सत्त्वशुद्धौ सौमनस्यैकाग्र्येन्द्रियजयात्मदर्शनयोग्यत्वानि च।

42. Santoṣādanuttamaḥ sukhalābhaḥ.
सन्तोषादनुत्तमः सुखलाभः।

43. Kāyendriyasiddhiraśuddhikṣayāttapasaḥ.
कायेन्द्रियसिद्धिरशुद्धिक्षयात्तपसः।

44. Svādhyāyādiṣṭadevatāsaṃprayogaḥ.
स्वाध्यायादिष्टदेवतासंप्रयोगः।

45. Samādhisiddhirīśvarapraṇidhānāt.
समाधिसिद्धिरीश्वरप्रणिधानात्।

46. Sthirasukhamāsanam.
स्थिरसुखमासनम्।

47. Prayatnaśaithilyānantasamāpattibhyām.
प्रयत्नशैथिल्यानन्तसमापत्तिभ्याम्।

48. Tato dvandvānabhighātaḥ.
ततो द्वन्द्वानभिघातः।

49. Tasmintsati śvāsapraśvāsayorgativicchedaḥ prāṇāyāmaḥ.
तस्मिन्सति श्वासप्रश्वासयोर्गतिविच्छेदः प्राणायामः।

50. Bāhyābhyantarastambhavṛttirdeśakāla-saṅkhyābhiḥ paridṛṣṭo dīrghasūkṣmaḥ.
बाह्याभ्यन्तरस्तम्भवृत्तिर्देशकालसंख्याभिः परिदृष्टो दीर्घसूक्ष्मः।

51. Bāhyābhyantaraviśayākṣepī caturthaḥ.
बाह्याभ्यन्तरविषयाक्षेपी चतुर्थः।

52. Tataḥ kṣīyate prakāśāvaraṇam.
ततः क्षीयते प्रकाशावरणम्।

53. Dhāraṇāsu ca yogyatā manasaḥ.
धारणासु च योग्यता मनसः।

54. Svaviśayāsaṃprayoge cittasya svarūpānukāra ivendriyāṇāṃ pratyāhāraḥ.
स्वविषयासंप्रयोगे चित्तस्य स्वरूपानुकार इवेन्द्रियाणां प्रत्याहारः।

55. Tataḥ paramāvaśyatendriyāṇāṃ.
ततः परमावश्यतेन्द्रियाणाम्।

CHAPTER - III

1. Deśabandhaṣcittasya dhāraṇā.
देशबन्धश्चित्तस्य धारणा।

2. Tatra pratyayaikatānatā dhyānam.
तत्र प्रत्ययैकतानता ध्यानम्।

3. Tadevārthamātranirbhāsaṃ svarūpaśūnyamiva samādhiḥ.
तदेवार्थमात्रनिर्भासं स्वरूपशून्यमिव समाधिः।

4. Trayamekatra saṃyamaḥ.
त्रयमेकत्र संयमः।

5. Tajjayāt prajñālokaḥ.
तज्जयात् प्रज्ञालोकः।

6. Tasya bhūmiṣu viniyogaḥ.
तस्य भूमिषु विनियोगः।

7. Trayamantaraṅgaṃ pūrvebhyaḥ.
त्रयमन्तरङ्गं पूर्वेभ्यः।

8. Tadapi bahiraṅgaṃ nirbījasya.
तदपि बहिरङ्गं निर्बीजस्य ।

9. Vyutthānanirodhasaṃskārayorabhibhavaprādurbhāvau nirodhakṣaṇacittānvayo nirodhapariṇāmaḥ.
व्युत्थाननिरोधसंस्कारयोरभिभवप्रादुर्भावौ निरोधक्षणचित्तान्वयो निरोधपरिणामः ।

10. Tasya praśāntavāhitā saṃskārāt.
तस्य प्रशान्तवाहिता संस्कारात् ।

11. Sarvārthataikāgratayoḥ kṣayodayau cittasya samādhipariṇāmaḥ.
सर्वार्थतैकाग्रतयोः क्षयोदयौ चित्तस्य समाधिपरिणामः ।

12. Tataḥ punaḥ śāntoditau tulyapratyayau cittasyaikāgratāpariṇāmaḥ.
ततः पुनः शान्तोदितौ तुल्यप्रत्ययौ चित्तस्यैकाग्रतापरिणामः ।

13. Etena bhūtendriyeṣu dharmalakṣaṇāvasthāpariṇāmā vyākhyātāḥ.
एतेन भूतेन्द्रियेषु धर्मलक्षणावस्थापरिणामा व्याख्याताः ।

14. Śāntoditāvyapadeśyadharmānupātī dharmī.
शान्तोदिताव्यपदेश्यधर्मानुपाती धर्मी ।

15. Kramānyatvaṃ pariṇāmānyatve hetuḥ.
क्रमान्यत्वं परिणामान्यत्वे हेतुः ।

16. Pariṇāmatrayasaṃyamādatītānāgatajñānam.
परिणामत्रयसंयमादतीतानागतज्ञानम् ।

17. Śabdārthapratyayānāmitaretarādhyāsātsaṅkarastat-pravibhāgasaṃyamāt sarvabhūtarutajñānam.
शब्दार्थप्रत्यायानामितरेतराध्यासात्सङ्करस्तत्प्रविभाग-संयमात्सर्वभूतरुतज्ञानम्।

18. Saṃskārasākṣātkaraṇāt pūrvajātijñānam.
संस्कारसाक्षात्करणात् पूर्वजातिज्ञानम्।

19. Pratyayasya paracittajñānam.
प्रत्ययस्य परचित्तज्ञानम्।

20. Kāyarūpasaṃyamāttadgrāhyaśaktistambhe cakṣuḥprakāśāsaṃprayoge' ntardhānam.
कायरूपसंयमात्तद्ग्राह्यशक्तिस्तम्भे चक्षु:प्रकाशासंप्रयोगेऽन्तर्धानम्।

21. Sopakramaṃ nirupakramaṃ ca karma tatsaṃyamādaparāntajñānamariṣṭebhyo vā.
सोपक्रमं निरुपक्रमं च कर्म तत्संयमादपरान्तज्ञानमरिष्टेभ्यो वा।

22. Maitryādiṣu balāni.
मैत्र्यादिषु बलानि।

23. Baleṣu hastibalādīni.
बलेषु हस्तिबलादीनि।

24. Pravṛttyā lokanyāsātsūkṣmavyavahita-viprakṛṣṭajñānam.
प्रवृत्त्या लोकन्यासात्सूक्ष्मव्यवहितविप्रकृष्टज्ञानम्।

25. Bhuvanajñānaṃ sūrye saṃyamāt.
भुवनज्ञानं सूर्ये संयमात्।

26. Candre tārāvyūhajñānam.
चन्द्रे ताराव्यूहज्ञानम्।

27. Dhruve tadgatijñānam.
ध्रुवे तद्गतिज्ञानम्।

28. Nābhicakre kāyavyūhajñānam.
नाभिचक्रे कायव्यूहज्ञानम्।

29. Kaṇṭhakūpe kṣutpipāsānivṛttiḥ.
कण्ठकूपे क्षुत्पिपासानिवृत्तिः।

30. Kūrmanāḍyāṃ sthairyam.
कूर्मनाड्यां स्थैर्यम्।

31. Mūrdhajyotiṣi siddhadarśanam.
मूर्धज्योतिषि सिद्धदर्शनम्।

32. Prātibhādvā sarvam.
प्रातिभाद्वा सर्वम्।

33. Hṛdaye cittasaṃvit.
हृदये चित्तसंवित्।

34. Sattvapuruṣayoratyantāsaṅkīrṇayoḥ pratyayāviśeṣo bhogaḥ parārthatvāt svārthasaṃyamāt puruṣajñānam.
सत्त्वपुरुषयोरत्यन्तासङ्कीर्णयोः प्रत्ययाविशेषो भोगः परार्थत्वात् स्वार्थसंयमात् पुरुषज्ञानम्।

35. Tataḥ prātibhaśrāvaṇavedanādarśāsvādavārtā jāyante.
ततः प्रातिभश्रावणवेदनादर्शास्वादवार्ता जायन्ते।

36. Te samādhāvupasargā vyutthāne siddhayaḥ.
ते समाधावुपसर्गा व्युत्थाने सिद्धयः।

37. Bandhakāraṇaśaithilyāt pracārasaṃvedanācca cittasya paraśarīrāveśaḥ.

बन्धकारणशैथिल्यात्प्रचारसंवेदनाच्च चित्तस्य परशरीरावेशः।

38. Udānajayājjalapaṅkakaṇṭakādiṣvasaṅga utkrāntiśca.

उदानजयाज्जलपङ्ककण्टकादिष्वसङ्ग उत्क्रान्तिश्च।

39. Samānajayājjvalanam.

समानजयाज्ज्वलनम्।

40. Śrotrākāśayoḥ sambandhasaṃyamāddivyaṃ śrotram.

श्रोत्राकाशयोः सम्बन्धसंयमाद्दिव्यं श्रोत्रम्।

41. Kāyākāśayoḥ sambandhasaṃyamāllaghutūlasamāpatteścākāśagamanam.

कायाकाशयोः सम्बन्धसंयमाल्लघुतूलसमापत्तेश्चाकाशगमनम्।

42. Bahirakalpitā vṛttirmahāvidehā tataḥ prakāśāvaraṇakṣayaḥ.

बहिरकल्पिता वृत्तिर्महाविदेहा ततः प्रकाशावरणक्षयः।

43. Sthūlasvarūpasūkṣmānvayārthavattvasaṃyamād bhūtajayaḥ.

स्थूलस्वरूपसूक्ष्मान्वयार्थवत्त्वसंयमाद् भूतजयः।

44. Tato' ṇimādiprādurbhāvaḥ kāyasampattaddharmānabhighātaśca.

ततोऽणिमादिप्रादुर्भावः कायसम्पत्तद्धर्मानभिघातश्च।

45. Rūpalāvaṇyabalavajrasaṃhananatvāni kāyasampat.

रूपलावण्यबलवज्रसंहननत्वानि कायसम्पत्।

46. Grahaṇasvarūpāsmitānvayārthavattvasaṃyamādin-driyajayaḥ.
ग्रहणस्वरूपास्मितान्वयार्थवत्त्वसंयमादिन्द्रियजयः।

47. Tato manojavitvaṃ vikaraṇabhāvaḥ pradhānajayaśca.
ततो मनोजवित्वं विकरणभावः प्रधानजयश्च।

48. Sattvapuruśānyatākhyātimātrasya sarvabhāvādhiṣṭhātṛtvaṃ sarvajñātṛtvaṃ ca.
सत्त्वपुरुषान्यताख्यातिमात्रस्य सर्वभावाधिष्ठातृत्वं सर्वज्ञातृत्वं च।

49. Tadvairāgyādapi doṣabījakśaye kaivalyam.
तद्वैराग्यादपि दोषबीजक्षये कैवल्यम्।

50. Sthānyupanimantraṇe saṇgasmayākaraṇaṃ punaraniṣṭaprasaṅgāt.
स्थान्युपनिमन्त्रणे सङ्गस्मयाकरणं पुनरनिष्टप्रसङ्गात्।

51. Kṣaṇatatkramayoḥ saṃyamād vivekajaṃ jñānam.
क्षणतत्क्रमयोः संयमाद्विवेकजं ज्ञानम्।

52. Jātilakṣaṇadeśairanyatānavacchedāt tulyayostataḥ pratipattiḥ.
जातिलक्षणदेशैरन्यतानवच्छेदात् तुल्ययोस्ततः प्रतिपत्तिः।

53. Tārakaṃ sarvaviṣayaṃ sarvathāviṣayamakramaṃ çeti vivekajajñānam.
तारकं सर्वविषयं सर्वथाविषयमक्रमं चेति विवेकजज्ञानम्।

54. Sattvapuruṣayoḥ śuddhisāmye kaivalyam.
सत्त्वपुरुषयोः शुद्धिसाम्ये कैवल्यम्।

CHAPTER - IV

1. Janmauṣadhimantratapaḥsamādhijāḥ siddhayaḥ.
जन्मौषधिमन्त्रतपःसमाधिजाः सिद्धयः।

2. Jātyantarapariṇāmaḥ prakṛtyāpūrāt.
जात्यन्तरपरिणामः प्रकृत्यापूरात्।

3. Nimittamaprayojakaṃ prakṛtīnāṃ varaṇabhedastu tataḥ kṣetrikavat.
निमित्तमप्रयोजकं प्रकृतीनां वरणभेदस्तु ततः क्षेत्रिकवत्।

4. Nirmāṇacittānyasmitāmātrat.
निर्माणचित्तान्यस्मितामात्रात्।

5. Pravṛttibhede prayojakaṃ cittamekamanekeṣām.
प्रवृत्तिभेदे प्रयोजकं चित्तमेकमनेकेषाम्।

6. Tatra dhyānajamanāśayam.
तत्र ध्यानजमनाशयम्।

7. Karmāśuklākṛṣṇaṃ yoginastrividhamitareṣām.
कर्माशुक्लाकृष्णं योगिनस्त्रिविधमितरेषाम्।

8. Tatastadvipākānuguṇānāmevābhivyak–tirvāsanānām.
ततस्तद्विपाकानुगुणानामेवाभिव्यक्तिर्वासनानाम्।

9. Jātideśakālavyavahitānāmapyānantaryaṃ smṛtisaṃskārayorekarūpatvāt.
जातिदेशकालव्यवहितानामप्यानन्तर्यं
स्मृतिसंस्कारयोरेकरूपत्वात्।

10. Tāsāmanāditvaṃ cāśiṣo nityatvāt.
तासामनादित्वं चाशिषो नित्यत्वात्।

11. Hetuphalāśrayālambanaiḥ saṅgṛhītatvādeṣāmabhāve tadabhāvaḥ.
हेतुफलाश्रयालम्बनैः संगृहीतत्वादेषामभावे तदभावः।

12. Atītānāgataṃ svarūpato'styadhvabhedāddharmāṇām.
अतीतानागतं स्वरूपतोऽस्त्यध्वभेदाद्धर्माणाम्।

13. Te vyaktasūkṣmā guṇātmānaḥ.
ते व्यक्तसूक्ष्मा गुणात्मानः।

14. Pariṇāmaikatvādvastutattvam.
परिणामैकत्वाद्वस्तुतत्त्वम्।

15. Vastusāmye cittabhedāttayorvibhaktaḥ panthāḥ.
वस्तुसाम्ये चित्तभेदात्तयोर्विभक्तः पन्थाः।

16. Na caikacittatantraṃ cedvastu tatpramāṇakaṃ tadā kiṃ syāt.
न चैकचित्ततन्त्रं चेद्वस्तु तत्प्रमाणकं तदा किं स्यात्।

17. Taduparāgāpekṣitvāccittasya vastu jñātājñātam.
तदुपरागापेक्षित्वाच्चित्तस्य वस्तु ज्ञाताज्ञातम्।

18. Sadā jñātāścittavṛttayastatprabhoḥ puruṣasyāpariṇāmitvāt.
सदा ज्ञाताश्चित्तवृत्तयस्तत्प्रभोः पुरुषस्यापरिणामित्वात्।

19. Na tatsvābhāsaṃ dṛśyatvāt.
न तत्स्वाभासं दृश्यत्वात्।

20. Ekasamaye cobhayānavadhāraṇam.
एकसमये चोभयानवधारणम्।

21. Cittāntaradṛśye buddhibuddheratiprasaṅgaḥ smṛtisaṅkaraśca.

चित्तान्तरदृश्ये बुद्धिबुद्धेरतिप्रसङ्गः स्मृतिसङ्करश्च।

22. Citterapratisaṅkramāyāstadākārāpattau svabuddhisaṃvedanam.

चित्तेरप्रतिसङ्क्रमायास्तदाकारापत्तौ स्वबुद्धिसंवेदनम्।

23. Draṣṭṛdṛśyoparaktaṃ cittaṃ sarvārtham.

द्रष्टृदृश्योपरक्तं चित्तं सर्वार्थम्।

24. Tadasaṅkhyeyavāsanābhiścittamapi parārthaṃ saṃhatyakāritvāt.

तदसङ्ख्येयवासनाभिश्चित्तमपि परार्थं संहत्यकारित्वात्।

25. Viśeṣadarśina ātmabhāvabhāvanāvinivṛttiḥ.

विशेषदर्शिन आत्मभावभावनाविनिवृत्तिः।

26. Tadā vivekanimnaṃ kaivalyaprāgbhāraṃ cittam.

तदा विवेकनिम्नं कैवल्यप्राग्भारं चित्तम्।

27. Tacchidreṣu pratyayāntarāṇi saṃskārebhyaḥ.

तच्छिद्रेषु प्रत्ययान्तराणि संस्कारेभ्यः।

28. Hānameṣāṃ kleśavaduktam.

हानमेषां क्लेशवदुक्तम्।

29. Prasaṅkhyāne' pyakusīdasya sarvathā vivekakhyāterdharmameghaḥ samādhiḥ.

प्रसङ्ख्यानेऽ प्यकुसीदस्य सर्वथा विवेकख्यातेर्धर्ममेघः समाधिः।

30. Tataḥ kleśakarmanivṛttiḥ.

ततः क्लेशकर्मनिवृत्तिः।

31. Tadā sarvāvaraṇamalāpetasya jñānasyānantyājjñeyamalpam.

तदा सर्वावरणमलापेतस्य ज्ञानस्यानन्त्याज्ज्ञेयमल्पम्।

32. Tataḥ kṛtārthānāṃ pariṇāmakramasamāptirguṇānām.

ततः कृतार्थानां परिणामक्रमसमाप्तिर्गुणानाम्।

33. Kṣaṇapratiyogī pariṇāmāparāntanirgrāhyaḥ kramaḥ.

क्षणप्रतियोगी परिणामापरान्तनिर्ग्राह्यः क्रमः।

34. Puruṣārthaśūnyānāṃ guṇānāṃ pratiprasavaḥ kaivalyaṃ svarūpapratiṣṭhā vā citiśaktiriti.

पुरुषार्थशून्यानां गुणानां प्रतिप्रसवः कैवल्यं स्वरूपप्रतिष्ठा वा चितिशक्तिरिति।

BIBLIOGRAPHY

- Buddha's Philosophy, The (G.F. Allen) (George Allen and Unwin Ltd., London)
- Buddhist Dictionary : Manual of Buddhist Terms and Doctrines (Nyanatiloka) (Frewin & Co., Ltd., Colombo, Ceylon)
- Dictionary of the Pali Language (Robert Caesar Childers) (Cosmo Publications, New Delhi)
- Early Buddhism and the Bhagavadgītā (K.N. Upadhyaya) (Motilal Banarsidass, Delhi - Varanasi - Patna)
- Gheranda Samhita (Srish Chandra Vasu) (Theosophical Publishing House, Adyar, Madras)
- Great Systems of Yoga (Ernst Wood) (D.B. Taraporevala Sons & Co. Pvt. Ltd., Bombay)
- Hathayoga Pradipika, The (Svatmarama) (The Theosophical Society, Adyar, Madras)
- Heyapaksha of Yoga, The (P.V. Pathak) (Asian Publication Services, New Delhi)
- History of Sanskrit Literature, A (A.B. Keith) (Oxford University Press, London E.C. 4)
- History of Yoga, A (Vivian Worthington) (Routledge & Kegan Paul, London)
- Importance of Vedanā and Sampajañña, The (Vipassana Research Institute, Igatpuri)
- Jataka Stories (E.B.Cowell) (Motilal Banarsidass Publishers Pvt. Ltd., Delhi)

- Jhānas in the Therāvāda Buddhist Meditation, The (Mahathera Henepola Gunaratana) (Buddhist Publication Society, Kandy, Sri-Lanka)
- Kundalini Yoga (Swami Sivananda) (Divine Life Society, Rishikesh)
- Mahāsatipaṭṭhāna Suttaṃ (Vipassana Research Institute, Igatpuri)
- Pali - English Dictionary (T.W. Rhys Davids & W. Stede) (Oriental Books Reprint Corporation, New Delhi)
- Patanjali's Yoga Sutras (Rama Prasada) (Munshiram Manoharlal Publishers Pvt. Ltd., New Delhi)
- Practical Yoga - Ancient and Modern (Ernst Wood) (Rider, London and Dutton, New York)
- Quintessence of Yoga Philosophy (D.V. Athalye) (D.B. Taraporevala Sons & Co. Pvt. Ltd.)
- Re-appraisal of Yoga, A (Georg Feuerstein & J. Miller) (Rider & Company, London)
- Sankara on the Yoga-sutras (Vol. I) (Trevor Leggette) (Routledge & Kegan Paul, London)
- Science of Yoga, The (I.K. Taimni) (Theosophical Publishing House, Adyar, Madras)
- Study of Patanjali, A (Surendranath Dasgupta) (University of Calcutta)
- Text-Book of Yoga (Georg Feuerstein)
- Time and Temporality in Samkhya Yoga and Abhidharma Buddhism (Brij Mohan Sinha) (Munshiram Manoharlal Publishers Pvt. Ltd., New Delhi)

- Visuddhimagga of Buddhaghosācariya (Henry Clarke Warren) (Harvard Oriental Series — Vol. XLI)
- Yoga (Ernst Wood) (Penguin Books Ltd., England)
- Yoga and Indian Philosophy (Karl Werner) (Motilal Banarsidass, Delhi-Varanasi-Patna)
- Yoga as Philosophy and Religion (Surendranath Dasgupta) (Motilal Banarsidass, Delhi-Varanasi-Patna)
- Yoga - Immortality and Freedom (Willard R. Trask) (Routledge & Kegan Paul, London)
- Yoga of Patanjali, The (M.R. Yardi) (Bhandarkar Oriental Research Institute, Pune)
- Yoga Stories and Parables (Swami Jyotirmayananda) (Miami, Florida, U.S.A)
- Yoga-Sutras of Patanjali (J.R. Ballantyne & Govind Sastri Deva)
- Yoga Sutras of Patanjali (M.N. Dwivedi) (Theosophical Publishing House, Adyar, Madras)
- Yoga-Sutras of Patanjali on Concentration of Mind, The (Fernando Tola & Carmen Dragonetti) (Tr. K.D. Prithipaul) (Motilal Banarsidass, Delhi)
- Yoga-System of Patanjali, The (James Haughton Woods) (Harvard Oriental Series, Vol. XVII)
- Yogavārttika of Vijñānabhikṣu (T.S. Rukmani) (Munshiram Manoharlal Publishers Pvt. Ltd., New Delhi)

- कल्याण योगाङ्क (भाग १० - अङ्क १,२,३)
(गीता प्रेस, गोरखपुर)

- पञ्चतन्त्र (विष्णुशर्मा)

- पातञ्जलयोगदर्शनम्
(श्रीनारायण मिश्र) (भारतीय विद्या प्रकाशन, वाराणसी)

- पातञ्जल योग प्रदीप
(स्वामी ओमानन्द तीर्थ) (गीता प्रेस, गोरखपुर)

- पातञ्जल योगशास्त्र - एक अध्ययन
(डॉ. ब्रह्ममित्र अवस्थी) (इन्दु प्रकाशन, दिल्ली)

- भारत के महान योगी
(विश्वनाथ मुखर्जी) (अनुराग प्रकाशन, वाराणसी)

- महामुनि पतञ्जलि - भ्रांतियां और निराकरण
(वैद्य दामोदरप्रसाद शर्मा शास्त्री) (नीलकण्ठ कालोनी, इन्दौर)

- योग - मीमांसा
(स्वामी सत्यपति परिव्राजक) (आर्ष साहित्य प्रचार ट्रस्ट, खारी बावली, दिल्ली)

- योगसूत्रम्
(डॉ. सुरेशचन्द्र श्रीवास्तव) (संवित् प्रकाशन, इलाहाबाद)

- श्रीमद्भगवद्गीता (गीता प्रेस, गोरखपुर)

- सांख्यकारिका
(ईश्वरकृष्ण) (हरिदास संस्कृत ग्रन्थमाला, २४९, बनारस)

- 'पालि तिपिटक' के सारे ग्रंथ (नालंदा संस्करण)
- नेत्तिपकरण अट्ठकथा
- विभङ्ग अट्ठकथा (सम्मोहविनोदनी)
- अट्ठसालिनी (पी. वी. बापट तथा आर. डी. वाडेकर) (ओरियण्टल रिसर्च इंस्टीट्यूट, पूना)
- विसुद्धिमग्ग (संपादक-संशोधन : डॉ. रेवतधम्म) संपूर्णानंद संस्कृत विश्वविद्यालय, वाराणसी
- जयमङ्गलअट्ठगाथा

List of VRI Publications

English Publications

- Sayagyi U Ba Khin Journal Rs. 325/-
- Essence of Tipitaka by U Ko Lay Rs. 155/-
- The Art of Living by Bill Hart Rs. 100/-
- The Discourse Summaries Rs. 65/-
- Healing the Healer by Dr. Paul Fleischman Rs. 45/-
- Come People of the World Rs. 40/-
- Gotama the Buddha: His Life and His Teaching Rs. 47/-
- The Gracious Flow of Dharma Rs. 55/-
- Discourses on Satipaṭṭhāna Sutta Rs. 90/-
- The Wheel of Dhamma Rotates Rs. 850/-
- Vipassana : Its Relevance to the Present World Rs. 160/-
- Dharma: Its True Nature Rs. 122/-
- Vipassana : Addictions & Health (Seminar 1989) Rs. 115/-
- The Importance of Vedanā and Sampajañña Rs. 165/-
- Pagoda Seminar, Oct. 1997 Rs. 80/
- Pagoda Souvenir, Oct. 1997 Rs. 50/-
- A Re-appraisal of Patanjali's Yoga- Sutra by S. N. Tandon Rs. 96/-
- The Manuals Of Dhamma by Ven. Ledi Sayadaw Rs. 280/-
- Was the Buddha a Pessimist? Rs. 65/-
- Psychological Effects of Vipassana on Tihar Jail Inmates Rs. 80/-
- Effect of Vipassana Meditation on Quality of Life (Tihar Jail) Rs. 100/-
- For the Benefit of Many Rs. 170/-
- Manual of Vipassana Meditation Rs. 85/-
- Realising Change Rs. 160/-
- The Clock of Vipassana Has Struck Rs. 167/-
- Meditation Now : Inner Peace through Inner Wisdom Rs. 90/-
- S. N. Goenka at the United Nations Rs. 25/-
- Defence Against External Invasion Rs. 10/-
- How to Defend the Republic? Rs. 6/-
- Why Was the Sakyan Republic Destroyed? Rs. 12/-
- Mahāsatipaṭṭhāna Sutta Rs. 70/-
- Pali Primer Rs. 95/-
- Key to Pali Primer Rs. 55/-
- Guidelines for the Practice of Vipassana Rs. 02/-
- Vipassana In Government Rs. 01/-
- The Caravan of Dhamma Rs. 90/-
- Peace Within Oneself Rs. 30/-
- The Global Pagoda Souvenir 29 Oct.2006 (English & Hindi) Rs. 60/-
- The Gem Set In Gold Rs. 145/-
- The Buddha's Non-Sectarian Teaching Rs. 15/-
- Acharya S. N. Goenka : An Introduction Rs. 35/-
- Value Inculcation through Self-Observation Rs. 55/-
- Pilgrimage to the Sacred Land of Dhamma (Hard Bound) Rs. 750/-
- An Ancient Path Rs. 120/-
- Vipassana Meditation and the Scientific World View Rs. 30/-
- Path of Joy Rs. 200/-
- The Great Buddha's Noble Teachings The Origin & Spreadof Vipassana (Small) Rs. 195/-
- Vipassana Meditation and Its Relevance to the World (Coffee Table Book) Rs. 800/-
- The Great Buddha's Noble Teachings The Origin & Spread of Vipassana (HB) Rs. 650/-
- Chronicles Of Dhamma Rs. 260/-
- Views on Vipassana Rs. 70/-
- Be Happy! (A Life Story of Meditation Teacher S.N.Goenka) Rs. 165/-
- Buddhaguṇagāthāvalī (in three scripts) Rs. 30/-
- Buddhasahassanāmāvalī (in seven scripts) Rs. 15/-
- English Pamphlets, Set of 9 Rs. 11/-
- Set of 12 Post Cards Rs. 35/-

Hindi Publications

- Nirmal Dhara Dharm Ki Rs. 65/-
- Pravachan Saransh Rs. 45/-
- Jage Pavan Prerana Rs. 90/-
- Jage Antarbodh Rs. 85/-
- Dharma: Adarsh Jivan ka Adhar Rs. 45/-
- Dharan Kare To Dharma Rs. 80/-
- Kya Buddha Dukhavadi The Rs. 45/-
- Mangal Jage Grihi Jivan Men Rs. 50/-
- Dhammavani Sangraha Rs. 45/-
- Vipassana Pagoda Smarika Rs. 100/-
- Suttasar-1 (Digha-Nikāya and Majjhima-Nikāya) Rs. 95/-
- Suttasar-2 (Samyutta-Nikāya) Rs. 90/-
- Suttasar-3 (Anguttara-Nikāya and Khuddaka-Nikāya) Rs. 80/-
- Dhanya Baba Rs. 58/-
- Kalyanamitra S. N. Goenka (Vyaktitva AurKrititva) by Mr. B. K. Goenka Rs. 50/-

- Patanjal Yoga Sutra by Shri Satyendranath Tandon Rs. 60/-
- Ahuneyya, Pahuneyya, Anjalikarniya Dr. Om Prakashji Rs. 40/-
- Rajdharm [Some Historical Events] Rs. 45/-
- Atma-Kathan, Part-1 Rs. 50/-
- Lok Guru Buddha Rs.10/-
- Desh Ki Bahya Surksha Rs. 05/-
- Ganrajya Ki Suraksha Kaise Ho! Rs. 06/-
- Shakyon Aur Koliyon Ke Gantantra Ka Vinash Kyo Huva? Rs. 10/-
- Aṅguttara Nikāya, Part I (Hindi Anuvad) Rs. 125/-
- Kendriy Karagrih Jaipur Rs. 50/-
- Vipassana Lokamat Part 1 Rs. 55/-
- Vipassana Lokamat Part 2 Rs. 70/-
- Agrapal Rajvaidya Jivaka Rs. 30/-
- Mangal Hua Prabhat (Hindi Dohe) Rs. 120/-
- Path Pradarshika Rs. 02/-
- Vipashyana Kyon Rs. 01/-
- Samrat Ashok Ke Abhilekh Rs. 70/-
- Pramukha Vipashyanacharya Shri Satya Narayan Goenka ka Sankshipta Jivan-Parichaya Rs. 30/-
- Ahinsa Kise Kahen Rs. 25/-
- Lakundaka Bhaddiya Rs. 10/-
- Gautam Buddha: Jivan Parichaya aur Shiksha Rs. 25/-
- Bhagvan Buddha ki Sampradāyiktāvihīn Shikshā Rs. 15/-
- Buddhajivan Chitravali Rs. 330/-
- Bhagavan Buddha ke Agrasravak Mahamoggalan Rs. 45/-
- Kya Buddha Nastik The Rs. 100/-
- Mahamanav Buddhanchi Mahan Vidya Vipassana: Ugama Ani Vikas (Big) (Hard Bound) Rs. 625/-
- Tip. Men Samyaka Sambuddha-(6 Parts) Part-1 Rs. 65/-, Part-2 Rs. 85/-, Part-3 Rs. 90/- Part-4 Rs. 75/-, Part-5 Rs. 80/-, Part-6 Rs. 85/-
- Bhagavan Buddha ke Mahasravak Mahamkassapa Rs. 40/-
- Mahamanav Buddha ki Mahan Vidya Vipassana ka Udgama Aur Vikas(Small Book) Rs. 145/-
- Bhagavan Buddha ke Agraupasak Anathapindika Rs. 50/-
- Bhagavan Buddha ke Agrasravika Kisagotmi Rs. 30/-
- Chitta Grihapati and hatthaka Alavaka Rs. 35/-
- Khushiyo Ki Rah Rs. 150/-
- Visakha Migaramata Rs. 45/-
- Magadharaja Seniya Bimbisara Rs. 55/-
- Buddhasahassanāmāvalī (Pali-Hindi) Rs. 35/-
- Ananda - Bhagwan Buddha ke Upasthak Rs. 130/-
- Jine ki kala Rs. 70/-
- Param Tapsvi Shri Ramsinghji Rs. 55/-
- Bhagwan Buddha Ki Agra-upasikayen Khujjuttara Evam Samavati Tatha Uttaranandmata Rs. 25/-
- Vipasyana Patrika Sangraha Part 1 Rs. 80/-
- Vipasyana Patrika Sangraha Part 2 Rs. 75/-
- Adarsa Dampati Nakulpita and Nakulmata Rs. 25/-
- Tikapaṭṭhān (Sankshipta Ruparekha) Rs. 35/-
- Bhagavan Buddha ke Agrasravaka Sariputta Rs. 65/-
- Burma men likhi Gayi Meri Kavitayaen Rs. 300/-
- Bāhiya Dārucīriya evaṃ Kuṇḍalakesā Rs. 30/-
- Rāhula evaṃ Raṭṭhapāla Rs. 40/-
- Puṇṇa Mantāṇiputta evaṃ Dhammadinnā Rs. 30/-
- Soṇa Koḷivisa evaṃ Soṇā Rs. 30/-
- Rahulmātā (Yashodharā) Rs. 35/-
- Bhagavana Buddha ke Mahāsrāvaka Ayushamān Aniruddha Rs. 35/-
- Vipasyana Patrika Sangraha Part 3 Rs. 74/-
- Vipasyana Patrika Sangraha Part 4 Rs. 84/-
- Khemā and Uppalavaṇṇā Rs. 30/-
- Paṭācārā and Bhaddā Kāpilānī Rs. 30/-
- Set of 12 Hindi Pamphlets Rs. 14/-
- Dhamma Vandana (Pali-Hindi) Rs. 45/-
- Dhammapada (Pali-Hindi) Rs. 45/-
- Mahāsatipaṭṭhānasutta (Bhasanuvad and Samiksha) (Pali-Hindi) Rs. 55/-
- Mahāsatipaṭṭhānasutta (Bhasanuvad) Rs. 35/-
- Prarambhik Pali (Pali Primer ka hindi anuvad) Rs. 85/-
- Prarambhik Pali ki Kunji (Key to Pali Primer ka hindi anuvad) Rs. 50/-
- Vishva Vipassana Stup ka Sandesh (Hindi, Marathi, English) Rs. 15/-

Rajasthani Publications

- Jago Loga Jagat Ra (Dohe) Rs. 45/-
- Paribhasha Dharam Ri Rs. 10/-
- Set of 5 Rajasthani Pamphlets Rs. 05/-

Marathi Publications

- Jaganyachi Kala Rs. 75/-
- Jage Pavan Prerana Rs. 80/-
- Pravachan Saransh Rs. 45/-
- Dharma: Aadarsh Jivanacha Aadhar Rs. 45/-
- Jage Antarbodh Rs. 65/-
- Nirmal Dhara Dharm Ki Rs. 45/-
- Mahāsatipaṭṭhānasutta (Bhasanuvad) Rs. 45/-
- Mahāsatipaṭṭhānasutta (Samiksha) Rs. 40/-
- Mangal Jage Grihi Jivan Mein Rs. 40/-
- Bhagavan Buddhachi Sampradayiktavihin Shikavanuk Rs. 12/-
- Buddhajivan Chitravali Rs. 330/-
- Anandachya Vatevar Rs. 150/-
- Atma-Kathan, Part-1 Rs. 50/-
- Agrapal Rajvaidya Jivaka Rs. 20/-
- Mahamanav Buddhanchi Mahan Vidya Vipassana: Ugama Ani Vikas (Small) Rs. 125/-
- Lok Guru Buddha Rs. 10/-
- Lakuṇḍaka Bhaddiya Rs. 12/-
- Pramukha Vipashyanacharya Satyanarayan Goenka Yancha Sankshipta Jivan-Parichaya Rs. 25/-
- Bhagavan Buddha ke Agraupasak Anathapindika Rs. 45/-
- Visakha Migaramata Rs. 35/-
- Chitta Grihapati and hatthaka Alavaka Rs. 30/-
- Bhagavan Buddha kee Agrasravika Kisagotmi Rs. 25/-
- Dhammapada (Pali-Marathi) Rs. 45/-
- Vipashyana Kaśāsāṭhī Rs. 01/-
- Magadharāja Seniya Bimbisāra Rs. 50/-
- Mahamanav Buddhanchi Mahan Vidya Vipassana: Ugama Ani Vikas Rs. 525/-
- Prarambhik Pali (Pali Primer ka Marathi anuvad) Rs. 65/-
- Prarambhik Pali ki Kunji (Key to Pali Primer ka Marathi anuvad) Rs. 40/-
- Bhagavan Buddha ke Mahasravak Mahamkassapa Rs. 35/-
- Bhagavan Buddha ke Agrasravak Mahamoggalan Rs. 45/-
- Kya Buddha Dukhavadi The Rs. 40/-

Gujarati Publications

- Pravachan Saransh Rs. 45/-
- Dharma: Aadarsh Jivanano Aadhar Rs. 50/-
- Mahāsatipaṭṭhānasutta Rs. 20/-
- Jage Antarbodh Rs. 85/-
- Dharan Kare To Dharma Rs. 80/-
- Jage Pavan Prerana Rs. 100/-
- Kya Buddha Dukhavadi The Rs. 40/-
- Vipassana Sha Mate Rs. 02/-
- Mangal Jage Grihi Jivan Men Rs. 40/-
- Nirmal Dhara Dharm Ki Rs. 70/-
- Buddhajivan Chitravali Rs. 330/-
- Lok Guru Buddha Rs. 06/-
- Bhagvan Buddha ki Sampradayiktavihin Shiksha Rs. 10/-
- Samrat Ashok ke Abhilekh Rs. 75/-

Other Publications

- The Art of Living (Tamil) Rs. 90/-
- Discourse Summaries (Tamil) Rs. 30/-
- Gracious Flow of Dhamma (Tamil) Rs. 55/-
- Mangal Jage Grihi Jivan Men (Telugu) Rs. 55/-
- Pravachan Saransh (Bengali) Rs. 65/-
- Dharma: Adarsh Jivan ka Adhar (Bengali) Rs. 60/-
- Mahāsatipaṭṭhānasutta (Bengali) Rs. 90/-
- Pravachan Saransh (Malayalam) Rs. 45/-
- Nirmal Dhara Dharm Ki (Malayalam) Rs. 45/-
- Jine ka Hunar (Urdu) Rs. 75/-
- Dharma: Adarsh Jivan ka Adhar (Punjabi) Rs. 50/-
- Nirmal Dhara Dharam Ki (Punjabi) Rs. 70/-
- Mangal Jage Grihi Jivan Mein (Punjabi) Rs. 50/-
- Kisagotmi (Punjabi) Rs. 30/-
- Gotama the Buddha: His Life and His Teaching (French) Rs. 50/-
- Meditation Now: Inner Peace through Inner Wisdom (French) Rs. 80/-
- For the Benefit of Many (French) Rs. 195/-
- For the Benefit of Many (Spanish) Rs. 190/-
- The Art of Living (Spanish) Rs. 130/-
- Path of Joy (German, Italian, Spanish, French) Rs. 300/-

Pali Publication

Aṅguttara Nikāya (PB) (12 vol.) Rs. 1500/-

Khuddaka Nikāya set-1 (9 vol.) Rs. 5400/-

Dīghanikāya Abhinava Tīka (Roman) (vol. I & II) Rs. 1000/-

For more information write to: Vipassana Research Institute, Dhamma Giri, Igatpuri 422 403, Maharashtra, India. Tel: [91] (02553) 244076, 244086, 243712, 243238; Fax: 244176, Email: vri_admin@dhamma.net.in; Website: www.vridhamma.org

You can purchase VRI publications ONLINE also. Please visit www.vridhamma.org

Vipassana Meditation Centres

There are 84 Vipassana centres in India and 94 centres in other countries of the world. The names of some centres are given below where 10-day courses are held every month. Those desirous of joining meditation course should seek information from any of the centres according to their convenience. visit:- <www.vridhamma.org> and www.dhamma.org

India

Maharashtra

Dhamma Giri, Dhamma Tapovana I and II, Vipassana International Academy, 422 403 Dist. Nashik, Tel: [91] (02553) 244076, 244086; Fax: [91] (02553) 244176; Website: www.vridhamma.org Email: info@giri.dhamma.org

Dhamma Pattana, Global Vipassana Pagoda, Near Essel World, Gorai Creek, Borivali (W), Mumbai 400 091. Tel: (022) 2845 2261, Tel/Fax: (022) 2845-2111, 2845 2112; Website: www.globalpagoda.org Course applications to: Manager, Dhamma Pattana, Near Essel World, Gorai Creek, Borivali (W), Mumbai 400091, Tel: (022) 2845-2238, 3374-7501, Mob. 97730-69975, Tel/Fax: (022) 3374-7531, Email: info@pattana.dhamma.org Website: www.pattana.dhamma.org;

Dhamma Thalī, Rajasthan Vipassana Centre, Via Sisodiya Rani Baug, Through Galtaji Road, Jaipur 302 001, Rajasthan Tel: [91] (0141) 2680 220, 2680 311, Email: info@thali.dhamma.org, Mob. 0-9610401401, 9982049732,

Dhamma Sindhu, Kutch Vipassana Centre, Village-Bada, Tal. Mandvi, Dist. Kutch 370 475 Tel: Off. [91] (02834) 273 303, **City Contact:** Tel. Res. (02834) 223 406; Off. 223 076, Mob. 99254-85981; Email: info@sindhu.dhamma.org

Dhamma Khetta, Vipassana International Meditation Centre, Kusumnagar, (12.6 km) Nagarjun Sagar Road, Vanasthali Puram, Hyderabad 500 070, A.P. Tel: Off. (040) 2424 0290, Fax: 2424 1746; City Off. 2473 2569, Email: info@khetta.dhamma.org

Dharmashringa, Nepal Vipassana Centre, PO. Box No. 12896, Budhanilkanth, Muhan Pokhari, Kathmandu, Nepal. Tel: [977] (01) 4371 655, 4371 007, City Contact: Tel: [977] (01) 4250 581, 4225 490; Email: info@shringa.dhamma.org;

Myanmar

Dhamma Joti, Vipassana Centre, Wingaba Yele Kyaung, Nga Htat Gyi Pagoda Road, Bahan, Yangon, Myanmar Tel: [95] (1) 549 290, 546660; Office: No. 77, Shwe Bon Tha Street, Yangon, Myanmar. Fax: [95] (1) 248 174 **Contact:** Mr. Banwari Goenka, Goenka Geha, 77 Shwe Bon Tha Street, Yangon, Myanmar Tel: [95] (1) 241708, 253601, 245201; Res. Mobile: 95950-13929; Email: bandoola@mptmail.net.mm; dhammajoti@mptmail.net.mm

Sri Lanka

Dhamma Kūṭa, Vipassana Meditation Centre, Mowbray, Hindagala, Peradeniya, Sri Lanka Tel: [94] (060) 280 0057; Email: dhamma@sltnet.lk

Thailand,

Dhamma Kamala, Thailand Vipassana Centre, 200 Yoo Pha Suk Road, Ban Nuen Pha Suk, Tambon Dong Khi Lek, Muang District, Prachinburi Province, 25000, Thailand Tel. [66] (037) 403- 514-6, [66] (037) 403 185; Email: info@kamala.dhamma.org

Australia & New Zealand,

Dhamma Bhūmi, Vipassana Centre, P. O. Box 103, Blackheath, NSW 2785, Australia Tel: [61] (02) 4787 7436; Fax: [61] (02) 4787 7221 Email: info@bhumi.dhamma.org

Europe,

Dhamma Dīpa, Harewood End, Herefordshire, HR2 8JS, UK Tel: [44] (01989) 730 234; Website: www.dipa.dhamma.org Email: info@dipa.dhamma.org

North America

Dhamma Dharā, VMC, 386 Colrain-Shelburne Road, Shelburne MA 01370-9672, USA Tel: [1] (413) 625 2160; Fax: [1] (413) 625 2170; Website: www.dhara.dhamma.org Email: info@dhara.dhamma.org

South Africa

Dhamma Patākā, (Rustig) Brandwacht, Worcester, 6850, P. O. Box 1771, Worcester 6849, South Africa Tel: [27] (23) 347 5446; Contact: Ms. Shanti Mather, Tel/Fax: [27] (028) 423 3449; Website: www.pataka.dhamma.org, Email: info@pataka.dhamma.org

For details like address, Phone no. and email of the rest of Vipassana centres, visit:- <www.vridhamma.org> and <www.dhamma.org>